Fruit & Vegetable Bible

For Juices, Smoothies and Natural Goodness

By Andrew J. Williams, Ph.D.

Version 1.4

Updated 27th October 2014

Contents

DISCLAIMER AND TERMS OF USE AGREEMENT

Introduction

Over the last few decades, we have been told what we should eat, and how much. Government guidelines have given us daily recommended amounts for each vitamin, mineral and macronutrient. Common advice around the world seems to be to eat more fruit and vegetables and whole-grains. We are also typically told to eat less salt, less saturated fats, sugars and refined grains. However, despite what they clearly see as an attempt to help, obesity, diabetes, heart disease, mental disorders, and disease in general, are at an all time high.

I really believe that the main cause of so many health problems stem from this advice, especially the "whole grains" and fats bit. However, that is for another book.

If we subscribe to the old adage "we are what we eat", then clearly the guidelines are not working. Our bodies are well-tuned machines that require a range of nutrients to function properly. When we don't give our body what it needs, it stops working efficiently, in exactly the same way as a car would if you stopped changing the oil, or giving it the correct fuel.

The ironic thing is that obesity and the other diseases we are currently facing in epidemic proportions were a lot rarer before the guidelines came in.

If we just look at the last 20 years, the stats are astonishing.

In 1995 – 1997, new diagnosis of type 2 diabetes was at the rate of 4.8 per 1000 people. By 2005 – 2007, that had risen to 9.1 per 1000 people. That's double the rate in 10 years[1].

If we look at obesity, the stats are just as frightening. In the past 30 years, obesity rates in the US have more than doubled, from 15 percent in 1976 – 1980, to 35.7 percent in 2009 – 2010. Compared to 1960, the average American is 24 pounds heavier[2].

Over the years, processed foods and GMO foods have found their way onto our tables. Fast food restaurants have made eating easy. With our busy lives, it's much easier to pop into a fast food "restaurant" and buy something that is undoubtedly delicious, or stop off at the supermarket and buy ready-made meals.

The problems with so many of these fast food solutions, is lack of quality nutrients. There is also the matter of additives, preservatives, colourings and flavourings. You would not be happy putting a lot of these chemicals into food you cooked at home, but you are quite happy to buy food someone else has prepared using these chemicals.

I get it, you are in a hurry and don't have too much time to prepare food. However, if you don't start looking after your own health and eating the foods that nature provides, you will more than likely end up as one of the epidemic statistics!

Fortunately, the solution to so many health problems is right in front of your eyes. Fresh fruit and vegetables! And before you start thinking or food preparation times, let me stop you there.

Juicing machines and blenders are there to help.

Blenders are perhaps the easiest option, since you just fill them with fresh produce and hit a switch to create a nutritious, and often delicious smoothie. Juicing is a little more involved, and takes a little more effort, especially cleaning the machine after use.

There are those people that prefer blending because of the extra fibre it provides over juicing. However, I believe there is a place for both. The beauty of juicing is that you can consume cocktails containing the vitamin, mineral and phytonutrient contents of big piles of fruit and vegetables. Far more in fact than you could eat, or drink as a smoothie. For anyone coming off years of junk food abuse, juicing offers a quick way to replenish your body stores of vital nutrients. In fact, it's not uncommon for people to get an actual buzz or "high" when they start juicing. Their body finally has the nutrients it's been craving, and things start to work more efficiently.

So what exactly do you put into your juices and smoothies?

Well, that is why I put this book together. It contains information on a wide range of common fruit and vegetables. You'll learn a little about the historical

2

use of the produce, but also its nutritional value. Where there is medical research on the fruit or vegetable, I've tried to include that, with references so you can check out some of the research for yourself.

The truth is, nature's larder contains everything your body needs to thrive, maintain and repair itself. This is the same larder our ancestors ate from, and by returning to it (and turning your back on junk food), you will find your health and happiness return.

Make a commitment today. Buy a juicer or blender, and start on your new path to health, vitality and happiness.

This book lists fruit and vegetables in alphabetical order, so you can easily find everything.

For more juicing tips, advice & recipes, you can visit my site – http://juicingtherainbow.com

Resources:

[1] http://www.reuters.com/article/2008/10/30/us-diabetes-usa-idUSTRE49T7JJ20081030?feedType=RSS&feedName=healthNews

[2] http://fasinfat.org/obesity-rates-trends-overview/

Alfalfa Sprouts

Introduction to Alfalfa Sprouts

Alfalfa is a legume belonging to the pea family (Papilioaceae), species *Medicago sativa*, and the mostly commonly grown crop in the world. Due to the high quantities of protein found in it, it is employed as food for all types of farm animals. Stems, leaves and sprouts from the seeds are all used for human consumption.

Alfalfa has many other qualities that make it a highly valuable plant besides its nutritional content. Its nitrogen-fixing abilities make it great for crop rotation to revitalize soil for other crops. Planted in partnership with grasses, it prevents soil erosion. Dried alfalfa is pulverized into meal and added to poultry and livestock feed. It is an indirect source of honey as bees collect large amounts of nectar from its flowers. It is also deemed to be an insectary, a place where insects are nurtured. Since it shelters predatory and parasitic pests it offers protection to crops planted near it. The quick harvesting plant thrives throughout the year, regardless of the temperature or climate, all over the world.

Alfalfa sprouts (also commonly called alfalfa grass) are immature shoots derived from alfalfa seeds. They are usually consumed within four to seven days after germinating. They are thin thread-like, white structures with petite green tops. The germination process for human consumption requires just water, a jar and some seeds. Just one tablespoon of seeds produces almost three cups of sprouts. Being small in size, the crunchy sprouts are jam-packed with nutrients and have only eight calories with no fat in each cup.

History of Alfalfa Sprouts

Alfalfa has been cultivated as a forage plant since antiquity and is a native of Asia Minor and Caucasus Mountains. It was grown by the Greeks, Persians and the Romans. Lucerne, Lucerne grass, Chilean clover and buffalo grass are some of it other common names.

It is believed that the name alfalfa originated in medieval times from the Iranian language. It was known as *"aspastor"* or *"ispist"* before being altered to *"al-fac-facah"* in Arabic. The Arabic name translates into "father of all foods", a reference to its high nutritional value. The final change in the name after the plant was introduced to Spain. The Spanish, being horsemen valued the plant highly and considered it to be the best horse feed. They started by calling it *"alfalfez"* and finally it became alfalfa. The Spanish colonizers introduced alfalfa to the Americas and the name has remained unchanged ever since.

Health Benefits of Alfalfa Sprouts

Alfalfa has been utilized as a herbal medicine for more than fifteen hundred years. Chinese physicians used the baby alfalfa leaves as treatment for digestive tract disorders and kidneys. Ayurvedic medicine recommends alfalfa for the treatment of bad digestion. A cooling poultice was also produced from its seeds to treat boils.

Alfalfa sprouts are one of the most potent sources of phytoestrogens. These valuable substances from plant foods can help in cutting down the risk of heart disease, cancer and osteoporosis[1]. They may even be advantageous in decreasing symptoms of menopause. Dr. Michael T Murray author of *The Condensed Encyclopedia of Healing Foods* also states that alfalfa sprouts have substances called saponins, which play a role in lowering LDL (bad cholesterol) while increasing HDL (good cholesterol) and may enhance immunity. Saponins are also believed to enhance the immune system by augmenting the activity of T-lymphocytes and interferons, body's natural killing machines of harmful invaders. The anti-inflammatory features of saponins aid in lowering the inflammatory progression of arthritis and chronic inflammatory ailments.

Alfalfa sprouts are a potent source of dietary protein, which raw-food advocates turn to when seeking to replace traditional protein sources. The three grams of protein in each serving make alfalfa the most consistent raw source of this essential macronutrient. One serving also provides one gram of fibre, which is equivalent to 3% of an adult's daily requirement. People suffering from digestive problems like chronic constipation or diverticular disease can benefit greatly by including alfalfa sprouts in the daily diet. The high quantity of protein and fibre combined with no saturated fat, cholesterol or sugar and only eight calories in a 33-gram serving, make alfalfa sprouts the perfect diet food.

Other than aiding in lowering the bad cholesterol, alfalfa sprouts can help in averting and treating atherosclerosis (plaque build-up in arteries of the heart) leading to hardening of the arteries. This is a serious disease which can lead to fatal problems, so before embarking on an alfalfa supplemented diet, discuss with your doctor the best course of action. It is also believed that alfalfa sprouts can be used as a complementary treatment for type-2 diabetes as it has no sugar. The canavanine, an amino acid analogue found in alfalfa sprouts is recognized to be helpful in combating leukemia, fibrocystic breast tumors, colon and pancreatic cancers.

Nutritional Value of Alfalfa Sprouts

Alfalfa sprouts generally tend to be very rich in nutrients since they house most of the energy the plant needs to grow and develop. They have elevated quantities of vitamins A, B, C, E and K. Sprouts are among nature's most concentrated suppliers of vitamin K. Vitamin K is critical for optimal platelet function and it helps to inhibit excessive bleeding (check with your doctor if you are taking anticoagulants as vitamin K may hinder the drug's efficiency).

Alfalfa sprouts also contain free amino acids, organic acids, non-protein amino acids like canavinine, strachydrine, isoflavonoids, coumarins, saponins, in addition to steroids like b-sitosterol, stigamsterol, campeterol etc. Minerals like potassium for healthy muscles, calcium to build bones and magnesium along with chlorophyll and carotene are all part of the health benefiting nutritional make-up of alfalfa sprouts.

How to Use Alfalfa Sprouts

Alfalfa sprouts can be used in a number of ways. They can be incorporated into soups, sandwiches or salads. Sprouts may be consumed raw or blended into smoothies. Juice of sprouts is mild flavoured so it can easily be combined with other favourite juices to make a healthy, refreshing drink. A few quick ways of getting full benefit of alfalfa sprouts includes:

- Divide pita bread in half and separate into two parts. Chop up one tomato, ½ a cup of alfalfa sprouts and ½ a cup of lettuce, and mix all ingredients in a bowl. Season with your favourite salad dressing and stuff into the bread, for a hardy nutritious snack.
- Mix alfalfa sprouts with scrambled eggs immediately before serving.
- Toast alfalfa sprouts by spreading them on a cookie sheet and placing them in an oven for 1-2 minutes. This will give the sprouts a crispy texture while eliminating any bacteria that may be there. Sprouts prepared may be added to salads, wraps or sandwiches.

Growing your own sprouts

Alfalfa sprouts are easy to grow with a small quantity of seeds producing a lot of sprouts, approximately in a ratio of 1 to 7.

- Add one tablespoon of seeds into a large jar.
- Add enough water so it is approximately one inch above the seeds.
- Cover the jar with a cheese cloth and secure using a rubber band.
- Allow the seeds to soak overnight, draining the water in the morning.
- Rinse the seeds twice a day for the next 4 - 5 days, while keeping the jar away from direct sunlight.

Clinical Trials with Alfalfa Sprouts

Some preliminary studies indicate that alfalfa sprouts may be beneficial in helping to normalize serum cholesterol levels in patients suffering from type II hyperlipoproteinemia. Preparations of alfalfa extracts neutralize the cholesterol while it is still in the stomach and before it reaches the liver, in this way excreting it from the body without any harmful effects[2, 3].

Numerous trials have been carried out in laboratories which indicate that the plant estrogens in alfalfa might be helpful for menopausal women[4, 5].

In rats fed a disease-causing fungus, Alfalfa in the diet helped the rats to remove more of the fungus from their bodies. It is theorized that this happens because one of the saponins from alfalfa damages cell membranes of the fungi.

Resources

[1]The Condensed Encyclopedia of Healing Foods by Michael T. Murray

[2] Levy S. New product newswire. Drug Topics. 1999; 19:22.

[3] Dewey D. Cholestaid. NuPharma . January 1, 2001.

[4]Kurzer MS, Xu X. Dietary phytoestrogens. *Annu Rev Nutr* . 1997; 17: 353-381.

[5]De Leo V, Lanzetta D, Cazzavacca R, et al. Treatment of neurovegetative menopausal symptoms with phytotherapeutic agent [in Italian; English abstract]. *Minerva Ginecol* . 1998;50:207-211

Apples

The apple tree is a member of the Rosaceae family belonging to the genus Malus. It is related to almonds, pears, and apricots. The tree can reach heights of six to fifteen feet, depending on soil, weather conditions, and the variety. Flowers of the apple tree are pink-white in colour and have five petals. It is among the most commonly cultivated fruit trees on the planet, with over 7,500 recognised cultivars.

It is believed that apple trees originated in Asia where its distant relative *Malus sieversii* can still be found growing in the wild. Apples are referred to in mythology and associated with many cultures including Greek, Roman, Norse, Muslim, and Christian folklore. According to Norse mythology, magic apples keep people young forever. The story of Adam and Eve in the Bible is often associated with apples, even though apples are never specifically mentioned. Pomona, a Roman goddess, tended her orchards and presented gifts of apples to her favourite subjects as a reward for flattering acts.   In more recent history, Isaac Newton came up with the law of gravity after seeing an apple drop from a tree.

Different varieties of apples are bred for varying purposes. These include cooking, eating fresh, and for the production of cider and vinegar. Wild apples can be grown easily from seeds, but domestic varieties are usually propagated by grafting. In 2010, the apple genome was decoded, allowing for an enhanced understanding of how to control pest problems and selectively breed apples.

China is the largest grower of apples, producing more than thirty million tonnes in 2010. United States is the second largest apple producer adding over 6% to the world's production. Other major apple producers include Turkey, Italy, India, and Poland. There are many health benefits associated with the consumption of apples. They are sometimes labelled "nature's toothbrush" due to the belief that they clean teeth and help in massaging gums.

History of Apples

Theory has it that apples originated in central and southern part of China, as this area is home to the Malus species. Over the course of time, seeds were spread by birds in the entire Northern Hemisphere. Crab apples arose from these, bitter-fruiting varieties. It is also believed that the edible apple (*Malus domestica*) is a complicated hybrid arising out of the wild, primitive apple species.

Around 2500 BCE, apple cultivation was common in Persia and northern Mesopotamia. The apple trees not only provided culinary delights but were also admired for their ornamental beauty in the gardens of Persia. Wealthy citizens of ancient Rome and Greece enjoyed apples as a dessert and for use at banquets. With advanced horticultural knowledge, the Greeks understood grafting techniques and were able to propagate special varieties in their orchards. Theophrastus, a Greek writer, noted "Seedlings of . . . apples produce an inferior kind which is acid instead of sweet . . . and this is why men graft." The Roman writer, Pliny, detailed more than twenty varieties in his journal, *Natural History*. As the Roman Empire expanded, apple orchards were established throughout Europe and Britain.

In North America, apple orchards constituted an important portion of farms in the seventeenth and eighteenth centuries. They were cultivated mainly for the production of hard cider, which at that time was the drink of choice seeing as water was not considered safe to drink. The whole family enjoyed apple cider, and any surplus was used as barter for goods or services needed.

Health Benefits of Apples

Consumption of apples is associated with numerous health benefits, among them being the prevention of cancer and heart disease, sugar control, lowering of cholesterol, protection against inflammation, and assist in weight loss. The flavonoid phloridzin is only found in apples and is said to protect against osteoporosis in post-menopausal women and enhance bone density. Boron is another element found in apples which promotes bone strength. The phytonutrient quercetin, also found in apples, offers protection against Parkinson's and Alzheimer's diseases. Other phytonutrients found in apples include phenolic acids which protect the apples from attacks by fungus, bacteria and viruses, as well as providing antioxidant and anti-cancer benefits.

Antioxidant protection is important to human health because the free radicals produced in the human body are atoms with odd number of electrons. Electrons prefer to travel in pairs, so the odd numbered free radicals are on the look-out for electrons from cells within the body. When an free radicals takes electrons from a cell in the body, it changes the cell, and instead of having a permeable membrane that allows passage of food, oxygen and waste, the cell becomes rigid and starves to death. If the free radicals steal electrons from the cell's mitochondria, it shuts them down and again the cell dies. Cell death occurring in this way leads to aging and illnesses.

Apples also have pectin, the material responsible for allowing jelly to solidify. Pectin helps to decrease LDL, the bad cholesterol in the body, thus helping to prevent heart diseases. The high fibre content in apples stops the absorption of LDL in the colon. The dietary fibre gives a feeling of being full for longer durations, which helps dieters lose weight faster, and it helps diabetics to keep blood sugar levels stable. It is also believed that flavonoids such as quercetin and Naringin are found in apples, and these may be responsible for halting lung and breast cancers.

Nutritional Value of Apples

Apples are a favourite fruit for health and fitness conscious individuals. A rich source of antioxidants and phytonutrients, apples are a 'must eat' for optimal health. A medium sized apple, roughly three inches in diameter, has 95 calories. It also contains 4.4 grams of dietary fibre, which makes up 18% of daily recommended intake for women and 12% for men. It also provides 21 grams of carbohydrates, which aid in metabolising fats and enables the nervous system to work at optimal levels.

About 10% of an apple is made up of carbohydrates while another 4% constitutes vitamins and minerals. Over 80% of the fruit is water. Apples float because they have a lot of air trapped in them. Removing the apple peel and core eliminates half of the vitamin C and dietary fibre. The apple pips have a bitter taste and contain traces of cyanide, but not enough to cause any harm. However, if you are juicing a lot of apples for young children, I do recommend you core the apples first.

Apples have a large variety of vitamins including folates, niacin, pantothenic acid, pyridoxine, riboflavin, thiamin, vitamins A, C, E and K. Electrolytes found in apples include sodium and potassium while the minerals include calcium, iron, magnesium phosphorus, and zinc. Phyto-nutrients carotene-B, Cryptoxanthin-B, and Lutein-zeaxanthin also make up part of an apple's nutritional profile.

How to Use Apples

There are numerous ways to enjoy apples, starting with the old fashioned approach of just biting into a whole apple and working around the core.

Applesauce topped with cinnamon is one way to get all the nutrients apples have to offer, and whether one buys the grocery store variety or prepares it at home, it tastes great either way.

In addition to apple juice, apple cider is a traditional drink served in the holiday season at Thanksgiving and Christmas time.

Apple juice served hot or cold, mulled or spiced, is one of the best ways for young and old alike to drink the juice of apples. Apple cider can be used instead for those who savour something a little stronger. The varieties of apples that have a higher tannin and acid content are especially grown for cider production.

Apples make great additions to certain types of salads. They complement a wide variety of ingredients like pecans, walnuts, cheddar and gorgonzola cheese, as well as citrus and poppy seed vinaigrette. Apples can be preserved as jams, turned into a jelly, dried or cooked in sweet and savoury dishes, and made into a pies or compotes.

Apple Tips

To keep apples from turning brown in salads, lightly brush cut slices with lemon juice.

To stop whole peeled apples from becoming discoloured, add some peeled slices to cold water with a little salt added to it, and then place the whole peeled apples in the water.

Discolouration from aluminium utensils can be eliminated by boiling apple peels with the utensils in a large pot for a few minutes.

Clinical Trials with Apples:

Because apples have been enjoyed the world over since ancient times, there are obviously plenty of health benefits associated with them. Many studies have been carried out over the years to test these claims. According to one paper published in 2008, flavonoids in a diet reduce the risk of heart disease[1]. Other studies concluded that consuming quercetin, a flavonoid found in ample supply in apple peels, can aid in eliminating chronic inflammation which contributes to cardiovascular disease[2].

In a separate study, it was suggested that quercetin provided protection against such atmospheric pollutants like cigarette smoke. This is achieved by cutting down on the number of free radicals that are exposed in tissue[3]. Australian researchers found that consuming apples can lower the risk of asthma in people in their late twenties to early forties[4]. Another study carried out in 2000 by Butland et al[5] found that there was a definite link between lung function and the quantity of apples consumed in a week. Consumption of five or more apples a week showed a better overall lung function.

Apple juice plays a positive role in memory. It was found that mice consuming two to three cups of apple juice performed better in a maze with less oxidative brain damage[6]. It is thought that this is due to the large number and quantities of antioxidants available in apple juice, which prevents damage caused by free radicals. In humans, fruits like apples have been linked with a reduction in degenerate conditions like Alzheimer's[7].

Resources

[1]Tribolo, S. et al, (2008) Comparative effects of quercetin and its predominant human metabolites on adhesion molecule expression in activated human

vascular endothelial cells, Atherosclerosis, Vol. 197, Issue 1, Pages 50-56.

[2]Wach, A. et al (2007), Quercetin content in some food and herbal samples, Food Chemistry, Vol. 100 , Issue 2, Pages 699-704.

[3] http://news.bbc.co.uk/1/hi/health/610068.stm

[4]R.K Woods et al (2003) Food and Nutrient Intakes and Asthma Risk in Young Adults, American Journal of Clinical Nutrition, Vol. 78, Issue 3, Pages 414-421.

[5]B. K Butland et al (2000), Diet, Lung Function, and Lung Function Decline in a Cohort or 2512 Middle Aged Men, Thorax, Vol. 55, Issue 2, Pages 102-108.

[6]F. Tchantchou et al (2005), Apple Juice Concentrate Prevents Oxidative Damage and Impaired Maze Performance in Aged Mice, Journal of Alzheimer's Disease, Vol 8, Issue 3, Pages 283-287.

[7]Q. Dai et al (2006) Fruit and Vegetable Juices and Alzheimer's Disease: The *Kame* Project, The American Journal of Medicine, Vol. 119, Issue 9, Pages 751-759.

Asparagus

Asparagus is a member of the Asparagaceae family, originally the lily family. Other members of this family include: garlic, onions, turnips, and leeks. It is a hardy perennial plant with more than two hundred species known to exist all the way from Siberia to South Africa. Many of the species grown in Africa are used for ornamental purposes, providing tantalizing greenery in floral presentations,   while the most common garden variety *Asparagus officinalis* is cultivated for consumption. The name "asparagus" originates from the Greek word *asparagos* (originally the Persian *asparag*) meaning "sprout" or "shoot". The term *officinalis* means 'of the dispensary' in Latin, a reference to the medicinal properties of asparagus.

The wild asparagus usually has rather thin shoots, even thinner than a pencil, and it is significantly different than the variety found in the local grocery store. Selective breeding techniques have led to a variety with thicker shoots which contain more edible flesh. The ancient Greeks valued asparagus highly, but the Romans were the first cultivators of the vegetable.

Asparagus is grown by sowing the seeds in beds during early spring, and allowed to grow for one full year before harvesting. The new plants have compressed buds in the middle known as the crown, and many hanging roots. While green asparagus is the most commonly seen variety in the supermarkets, purple and white varieties also exist. The white asparagus is delicate and difficult to harvest, and the purple variety is smaller in size with a fruiter taste. Nutrition wise they are all very similar.

A carefully planted and cared for bed can continue to generate the vegetable for up to 20 years without the need to replant. The first plants are not usually harvested until three years old. This is to allow them to develop a strong fibrous root system. Once the harvesting is completed, the remaining spears develop into ferns, which then produce red berries that provide nutrients needed for the next year's crop.

Asparagus contains a distinctive compound which gives off a very characteristic smell in urine when metabolized. The younger shoots have a greater concentration of this sulphuric compound, and eating them gives an even stronger odour. While practically all people develop the odour in their urine after eating asparagus, most do not have the ability to detect it. No harmful effects arise due to the odour or the breakdown of the sulphuric compound.

History of Asparagus

According to most accounts, asparagus originated in the Middle East, where it still grows along the sand dunes and in river valleys. From here it spread into Europe and further west. Asparagus has a long history; it is believed that the Chinese were acquainted with the plant as far back as 4,000 years. Egyptians were growing asparagus more than 2,000 years ago, for its medicinal attributes. In fact, they valued it so highly that Pharaoh Ikhnaton and Nefertiti proclaimed it to be food of the gods, and so made offerings of asparagus in rituals to their deities.

There are records of Romans and Greeks growing asparagus in the first century. M. Porcius Cato, the Elder, wrote a detailed description of asparagus in his book 'De Agricultura' approximately 160 BCE. He described methods of growing the plant in home gardens, sowing times, duration, best ways to harvest the vegetable, weed control, and how to remove the dried fern from asparagus. They valued the vegetable for its distinctive flavour and supposed medicinal qualities. The Romans went so far as to start freezing the plant so that it could be enjoyed out of season. High-speed chariots and runners were employed to transport it to the snow laden Alps, where it stayed frozen until needed. Asparagus fleets guaranteed the delivery of the delicacy to all parts of the Empire.

Asparagus is pictured in murals found in Pompeii and was deemed to be a fine delicacy. Around the year 1100, Byzantine physicians declared asparagus as a medicinal plant for the first time, and derived the name *Asparagus officinalis*. The diuretic effect of the plant was employed to eliminate hip pains. At this time it was also considered to be an aphrodisiac and dedicated by the Romans to Venus, the goddess of love and beauty.

Asparagus was not used much during the middle ages but recaptured its popularity during the 16th century when it gained acceptance in Europe's royal courts. France's Louis XIV called asparagus the "king of vegetables" and ordered the construction of greenhouses so that he could enjoy it year-round.

In the 17th century, cultivation started in England where it was called sparrowgrass. Colonists carried it to the New World, where it was initially known by the same name.

Health Benefits of Asparagus

The medicinal value of *Asparagus officinalis* has been known since ancient Roman and Greek times. Dioscorides, a Greek physician in the first century, advocated asparagus root extracts for flushing out the kidney, jaundice, and sciatica. It was also referred to in the Gerard's Herbal for cleansing the system without causing dryness, increasing sperm, and to promote desires. In Ayurvedic medicine it is used in female infertility, and in Asian medicine it is given for diarrhoea, coughs, and nervous system issues.

In modern times, *Asparagus officinalis is* considered a strong diuretic and used for treating urinary problems like cystitis. It is also used in treating rheumatic problems, and also known to work as a gentle sedative and a laxative. Furthermore, it is beneficial in treating a number of ills, including arthrosis and tuberculosis.

The high content of glutathione found in asparagus is a strong antioxidant that is known to enhance the immune system, cut down inflammation, and preserve liver health. Glutathione breaks down carcinogens and free radicals which are responsible for causing cell damage, and also detoxifies the body. This is why it can be beneficial in fighting against certain cancers like bone, breast, larynx, and colon. The folate in asparagus works in conjunction with vitamin B12 to ward off cognitive decline. It also contains elevated levels of asparagines, an amino acid which serves as a natural diuretic helping to eliminate body's excess salts. This is particularly beneficial for people suffering from oedema (build-up of fluids in body tissues), and those with high blood pressure.

Nutritional Value Asparagus

Asparagus is a gold mine of nutrients that contribute to good health. Being a low calorie food, with only twenty calories in every 100 grams of fresh vegetable, it is the perfect complement to any weight loss program. In fact, most of those calories are burned off while digesting the vegetable itself. Out of the 100 grams, 2.1 grams make up dietary-fibre, which benefits ailments like constipation, regulating blood sugar, and lowering LDL (the bad cholesterol). A high fibre diet lowers the risks of colon-rectal cancer by putting an end to absorption of toxic compounds from food.

Asparagus spears are also a rich source of antioxidants like lutein, zeaxanthin, carotenes, and *cryptoxanthins*. The flavonoids help to eliminate the body of free radicals and possibly protect it against neuro-degenerative diseases, cancer, and viral infections. Asparagus also provides 14% of the RDA of folic acid. Folates are needed for DNA synthesis, and help to prevent neural tube defects in newborn babies.

Asparagus shoots are a good source of the B-complex vitamins like thiamine, riboflavin, niacin, pyridoxine and pantothenic acid. They also contain antioxidant vitamins like Vitamins C, A, and E. This group of vitamins help the body to build resistance against infectious diseases and remove harmful, inflammatory free-radicals. The ample amounts of vitamin K in asparagus promotes bone health, limits the brain neuron damage, and plays a positive role in patients with Alzheimer's disease.

Regular consumption of asparagus also supplies the body with important minerals like copper and iron, and trace amounts of calcium, manganese, potassium, and phosphorus. Copper is used in red blood production, and iron is needed for cell respiration and formation of red blood cells. Manganese is used as a co-factor for superoxide dismutase, an antioxidant enzyme. Potassium helps to control the heart rate and blood pressure by negating the effects of sodium.

How to Use Asparagus

To attain peak flavour, it is best to use asparagus at the time of purchase, as the spears begin to lose taste and moisture immediately after harvest. To prepare the vegetable, start by washing it with cool running water and trim roughly one inch off of the end (if you bend the asparagus, it usually breaks off where the shoot starts to become less woody). You can add the woody stems and peelings to cooking water. This makes the water quiet palatable and is great for using as a stock for soups.

Asparagus may be eaten raw, steamed, grilled, boiled, roasted, stir-fried, or even worked into casseroles and salads. The key to cooking asparagus perfectly is to "cook it briefly." Waterless methods of cooking are best for preserving the nutritional value and antioxidant power of the vegetable.

Asparagus blends well with a number of different ingredients, but it can be tasty on its own dressed with only lemon juice, olive oil, salt and pepper. It can be served raw as crudités with a dipping sauce. In a salads, it is best to hold the asparagus back until it's time to serve and then add it at the very last minute. Adding it too soon, will result in the high acidic content of salad dressings turning the spears an unsightly yellow. Fresh chives, thyme, tarragon, and savoury added to asparagus helps to enhance the flavour of its shoots.

Clinical Trials

While traditional Chinese and Korean medicine has used Asparagus cochinchinensis Merrill (ACE) as a treatment for inflammatory diseases, a 2009 published study showed ACE to be an effective anti-inflammatory agent and having therapeutic value against immune-linked cutaneous infections[1].

In another study published in 2006, it was found that plants like asparagus are a good source of anti-diabetic compounds. Extracts from asparagus helped to increase production of insulin. This can provide opportunities in new treatments for diabetic patients[2].

Resources

[1]http://www.ncbi.nlm.nih.gov/pubmed/18691647

[2]http://www.youtharia.com/clinical_studies/asparagus_adscendens

Basil Leaves

Introduction to basil leaves

Basil is a highly fragrant herb that is most commonly used for seasoning purposes. It is associated more with Mediterranean cooking but is also very common in Asian cuisine but is cultivated all over the world. It has become the most easily recognizable plant since pesto, a blend of basil, pine nuts and parmesan cheese gained popularity. There are over 60 kinds of basil and all differ from each other to some extent in taste and physical appearance. In appearance basil resembles peppermint a bit, which is understandable since they belong to the same family (lamiaceae).

Sweet basil (*Ocimum basilicum*), has forceful, sweet flavor and strong aroma, while the other varieties offer flavors that resemble their names: anise basil, lemon basil, and cinnamon basil. Holy basil (*Ocimum tenuiflorum*, also known as *Ocimum sanctum* and tulsi), is considered a holy plant in Hindu religious tradition and is worshiped in the mornings and evenings. The name 'tulsi' denotes "the incomparable one". The plant is considered to be a strong protector and is frequently planted around temples and placed with the dead. Basil is thought to be a love token and is planted on graves in Egypt, Iran and Malaysia.

The origin of basil's scientific name is partially explained by Greek mythology. Ocimus was responsible for organizing contests in honor of Pallas (ruler of Paralia or Diacria) and had fifty sons. It is claimed that when Ocimus was killed at the hands of a gladiator, basil appeared. The remaining part of the name is drawn from Medieval Latin form of the Greek word "*basileus*" meaning "King"

History of Basil

It is believed that basil's origins lie in the tropical areas of Thailand, Pakistan and India and has been cultivated there for over thousands of years. The first recorded account of basil probably goes back to its cultivation in Egypt, for possible use in embalming.

Basil has a very colorful history associated with it which dates as far back as the third century B.C.E. During the ancient times and up to the time basil was introduced to England somewhere near the 1500s, it was believed that crushed basil placed under a rock would give rise to serpents. Due to this legend, the common name of the herb comes from the Latin word "basilicum", a mythological giant of a serpent. It was further believed that if ingested, basil would make scorpions grow in the brain. Basil was taken to North America in the early 1600s.

During the Middle Ages medicine men of the times thought basil was poisonous. This was based on the fact that basil could not grow in the vicinity of Rue, a woody plant with strong smell and bitter flavor whose oil was used in medicines. Rue was believed to be poisonous to the enemy and anything that could not grow in its vicinity was naturally considered to be poisonous.

Health Benefits of Basil

Basil's extracts have been used to cure many ailments throughout history starting with simple problems like the common cold, stomach issues to more complex problems like heart disease, certain form of poisoning and malaria. Oils extracted from the plant are employed in manufacture of herbal toiletries. More recently basil has been found to be effective against a host of different ailments.

The Orientin and vicenin, two flavonoids found in basil protect cells and chromosomes from radiation and oxygen related damage. Additionally it protects against undesirable bacterial growth. Studies indicate that the explosive oil components in basil namely estragole, linalool, cineole, sabinene, eugenol, limonene and myrcene are responsible for inhibiting growth of pathogenic bacteria that no longer respond to the most commonly used antibiotic drugs[1, 2, 3].

Many over the counter anti-inflammatory medicines like asprin, ibuprofen and the frequently used acetaminophen work by inhibiting the function of the enzyme cyclooxygenase. The oil component eugenol blocks the very same enzyme. This ability to block the enzyme makes basil an anti-inflammatory herb capable of providing relief from conditions like rheumatoid arthritis and inflammatory bowel conditions.

Basil's high concentration of carotenoids like beta-carotene (also called "pro-vitamin A" because it gets converted to vitamin A) is a very powerful antioxidant which protects epithelial cells from damage caused by free radicals. It also keeps free radicals from oxidizing cholesterol in the blood vessels. Since cholesterol accumulates in the blood vessels only after it has been oxidized, basil averts the development of atherosclerosis which can lead to heart attack or stroke. Free radicals also contribute to ailments like osteoarthritis, asthma, and rheumatoid arthritis. The beta-carotene reduces the development of these diseases while halting further damage.

The magnesium in basil helps muscle and blood vessels to relax. This improves blood circulation and cut down on the risks of heart muscle spasms, and irregular heart rhythms. Other more traditional benefits of basil include it use as a diuretic to flush out kidneys, relief from flatulence and fullness.

Nutritional Value

Basil has very few calories and is a very low in saturated fats, cholesterol and sodium. It is a good source of protein, dietary fibre and many minerals and vitamins essential for good health. It is an outstanding source of Vitamin A, E, C, K, B6, Folate, Riboflavin and Niacin. It is also a very good source of minerals like Calcium, iron, magnesium, phosphorus, potassium, zinc, copper and manganese.

The various varieties of basil differ in their specific nutritional content, but the average Recommended Daily Value of some nutrients found in 100 grams of basil in general include:

- Iron: 40%
- Calcium: 18%
- Protein: 3 grams
- Vitamin A: 100%
- Vitamin K: 345%
- Vitamin C: 30%

Uses of basil

Being a herb, basil is most commonly used fresh in cooked foods. It is best when added at the very last stages of cooking, or used as garnish on top of a dish after it has finished cooking. This ensures that all nutrients remain intact and also over cooking basil destroys its flavor. The herb has refrigerator life of a few days, but it can be kept in a freezer for longer durations after blanching in boiling water very quickly. Although basil is commonly available in dried form, it loses most of its flavor in this form and what remains is quite different from the original fresh taste.

Everyone one is familiar with basil's use in pesto and its addition to tomato sauces. It is also great when combined with mozzarella and tomatoes sprinkled with olive oil for a traditional Caprese salad. It can be chopped or blended with soft butter and poured over steaks, roast chicken or boiled potatoes.

A few other unconventional ways to use basil include:

- Basil is proven to keep flies, mosquitoes and roaches away. Many chefs are known to keep basil plants in the kitchen to keep free from pests and fresh smelling.
- A number of basil varieties produce attractive flowers and buds. These stems look great when employed in flower arrangements.
- Basil provides a very appealing aroma when used in scented candles and soaps.
- It makes a great potpourri ingredient.
- Some varieties are very well suited for hedging and border purposes in gardens.

Clinical Trials

Basil has been the subject of numerous studies trying to establish how its nutritional components functions. While many of these studies are carried out *in vitro* and other on animals, its benefits to human ailments is gaining acceptance. Holy basil in particular contains powerful antioxidants and enjoys a safe GRAS status in the U.S. Clinical studies involving basil's effect on ulcers and controlling blood sugar levels in type II diabetics show some promise[4, 5].

In some initial clinical trials, asthma patients treated with five hundred milligrams of holy basil thrice daily, improved breathing and cut down on the frequency of attacks[7]. In another study carried out in Thailand, the effectiveness of three different varieties of basil leaf oils was tested for treatment of acne. It was found that oils from sweet basil and holy basil were effective against acne[5].

Resources

[1] Bozin B, Mimica-Dukic N, Simin N, Anackov G (March 2006). "Characterization of the volatile composition of essential oils of some lamiaceae spices and the antimicrobial and antioxidant activities of the entire oils". J. Agric. Food Chem. 54 (5): 1822-8. doi:10.1021/jf051922u. PMID 16506839.

[2] Chiang LC, Ng LT, Cheng PW, Chiang W, Lin CC (October 2005). "Antiviral activities of extracts and selected pure constituents of Ocimum basilicum". Clin. Exp. Pharmacol. Physiol. 32 (10): 811-6. doi:10.1111/j.1440-1681.2005.04270.x. PMID 16173941.

[3] de Almeida I, Alviano DS, Vieira DP, *et al.* (July 2007). "Antigiardial activity of Ocimum basilicum essential oil". *Parasitol. Res.* **101** (2): 443-52. doi:10.1007/s00436-007-0502-2. PMID 17342533.

[4] http://www.uofmhealth.org/health-library/hn-4597000#hn-4597000-uses

[5] Mountain Rose Herbs.com, "Holy Basil (Tulsi) Herb Profile"

http://www.mountainroseherbs.com/learn/Holy_basil.php

[6] http://www.healthline.com/natstandardcontent/holy-basil

[7] http://www.peacehealth.org/xhtml/content/cam/hn-4597000.html

Beets with Leaves & Stem

Introduction to Beets

Beets are also referred to as blood turnips and are members of a flowering plant belonging to the *Beta vulgaris* species. Beets are mainly cultivated for their roots but the green tops are edible also. There are nine other members of the Beta genus, all having the common name beet however *Beta vulgaris* is the most commercially important variety. The root provides ecological value by providing food for a variety of animals, and it holds commercial and important nutritional value for humans.

There are four major cultivar groups. The *garden beet* is mainly used as a vegetable whose roots and leaves are edible. The *sugar beet* is used for sugar production, the *mangel-wulzel* is grown as food for livestock and the *Swiss chard* is cultivated for its edible leaves. Approximately 30% of the world's production of sugar is derived from beets.

Beet roots are typically deep purple colour but white and golden varieties are also available. The leaves have a slightly bitter taste while the round root is sweet tasting. Due to the high level of sugar content in beets, they are very tasty even when consumed raw, but usually they are cooked or pickled.

The world's top Paralympic gold medallist, David Weir credits his success to drinking beet juice regularly. It is believed that nutrients in beets boost stamina. World's top commercial growers of beets include USA, Russia, Poland, Germany and France.

History of Beets

The beets we see today have evolved from wild sea-beet, a native along coasts from India all the way to Britain. The earliest recorded mention of beets is seen in the 8th century B.C.E in Mesopotamia. According to Roman and Jewish sources beets were already domesticated by the 1st century B.C.E. in the Mediterranean basin. It was the leaves of the very first domesticated varieties that were used for consumption. Remains of beet have been unearthed at the

3rd century Saqqara pyramid located at Thebes, Egypt, and burnt beets have also been discovered at a Neolithic site in the Netherlands. It is believed that the name of the vegetable is derived from the Greek letter beta, as the inflated root looks like the Greek B.

Romans cultivated beets intensely and their recipes included cooking beets with wine and honey. Apicius, a well-known gourmet of the times, used them in broths and even suggested using them in salads dressed with mustard, vinegar and oil in his book entitled "The Art of Cooking". Initially beets were more valued for their medicinal properties rather than for food value. They were used as treatment for fevers, wounds and various skin disorders, and constipation. In those days the beet root was longer and thin, resembling a carrot. The rounded shape more common now, did not come into existence until the 16th century.

Beet root grew in popularity during the Victorian times when it was used in cakes and puddings in addition to soups and salads. In the middle 1700s Andreas Marggraf, a German chemist identified sucrose in beets. Later one of his students constructed a sugar beet processing factory which was operational from 1801 until its destruction in the Napoleonic Wars. After World War II, the pickled forms of the vegetable were used most frequently. Beets were introduced to North America by the colonists, and were well established by the 18th century. George Washington is known to have used beets to carry out experiments at Mount Vernon.

Health Benefits of Beets & Stems

Root beets and their greens are a treasure trove of health benefiting nutrients with powerful antioxidant characteristics. Betacyanin is the pigment that gives beet root its rich colour, but more importantly it is an antioxidant. Antioxidants along with the carotenoids and flavonoids are believed to play a role in reducing the oxidation of LDL (bad cholesterol) and preventing its deposits in the arteries. This helps to protect the walls of blood vessels, and reduce blood pressure & cut down on heart attack risks. The betacyanin also helps to rid the body of dangerous toxins while averting development of cancerous tumors like leukemia, lung, colon, skin, breast, liver and prostate.

The carotenoids, zeaxanthin and lutein in raw beets aid in maintaining the health of the retina.

The folic acid in beet roots is necessary for normal tissue growth and the development of a baby's spinal cord. It also aids in preventing spinal cord defects like spina bifida. The iron is great for mothers to be also, as it provides an energy boost to mothers experiencing fatigue during pregnancy while preventing anaemia.

Silica in the beet root helps the body to fully absorb calcium, which is needed for healthy bones, thereby lowering the risks of osteoporosis. Even though beets contain a lot of sugar, it has almost no fat and few calories. Its low (2.9) Glycaemic Load means its conversion to sugars is very slow, thus making it a good candidate for keeping sugar levels stable. The high content of nitrates in beets helps to postpone progression of dementia. The nitric oxide produced in the blood upon consumption of beets helps to increase blood flow to the brain.

Beetroot was used as an aphrodisiac by ancient Romans. Science tells us that the high content of boron in beets is directly linked with human sex hormone production. Being a high fibre food, consumption of beets aids in digestion and colon cleansing. The oxalic acid in raw beets dilutes inorganic calcium remnants in the body. Remains of inorganic calcium are linked with many chronic diseases like arthritis, eye problems, arteriosclerosis, heart disease and kidney stones.

Nutritional Value of Beets & Greens

Each 100 gram serving of beetroot only has 38 kcal, but 1.7 grams of protein, 1.9 grams of fibre and 7.6 grams of carbohydrates. It has almost no fat (0.1g) and only 0.1 grams of sodium. The same one hundred gram serving provides 8% of the Recommended Daily Amount of vitamin C, 75% Folic Acid, 11% potassium, 7% iron, 3% zinc and 4% magnesium for the average adult women. A mere three baby beetroots provide one out of the five recommended portions of vegetables and fruit.

The greens of beets are a great source of carotenoids, flavonoids, antioxidants, and vitamin A. These compounds are found in greater quantities in the green than in the root of the beet. Vitamin A is needed for hearty mucus membranes, skin and good vision.

How to Use Beets

Prepare beets by rinsing them under cold water, while being careful not to tear the skin. Beet juice can stain the skin, so use gloves; if hands still get stained, then just rub lemon juice on the affected area to remove the stain. To ensure that you get the maximum nutritional benefits from beets, it is best not to over-cook them. Steaming the vegetable for fifteen minutes preserves their nutritional value and flavour.

Beets bleed quiet a bit when put in water. To limit bleeding and preserve maximum amounts of nutrients, it is best to leave at least 1 inch of the greens on top and the entire root intact. Then boil them whole and unpeeled. Once soft, remove from heat and allow them to cool sufficiently so they can be handled with ease. Now roots and if desired the stems too may be removed and the skin just rubbed off. In this condition they can be diced, chopped, sliced or even grated for use in desired recipes.

To roast beets, remove the greens and root and peel the beet. Next, slice them and place them in a roasting pan topped off with a light coating of oil. Sprinkle salt, dried thyme, oregano, and dill to taste and roast at 400° F for approximately 25 – 30 minutes. Other methods of cooking beets include steaming, sautéing, or just consuming raw.

Beet greens are not only edible but very healthy also. Greens should be prepared soon after purchase to gain full benefit of their nutrients. Wash the greens thoroughly under cold running water then chop coarsely. Place in a sauce pan with about half an inch of water. Greens cook down a lot so make sure you start with plenty of them! Squeeze the juice from one lemon in the cooking water and add salt to taste. Cook over high heat without cover, once the water is all evaporated and the greens soft, they are ready to be eaten.

Juicing beet roots is one of the best ways to get the full benefit of nutrients in this vegetable. Whether on their own or in combination with other ingredients, they provide a refreshing way to quench your thirst. Here is a great tasting recipe you should try.

Zesty Beet, Pineapple & Cucumber Juice

- 1 small beet root (may even use a couple of inches of the greens)
- 1 small cucumber
- 1 cup of pineapple pieces

Directions:

- Clean the beet root thoroughly, ensuring that all the dirt has been removed.
- If the cucumber is waxed, peel it, otherwise just wash it and it is ready for use.
- Remove the pineapple skin and chop into pieces, (only one cup is required, the remaining may be saved for later use.)
- Press all fruits through a juicer and serve chilled in tall glasses.

Clinical Trials

There are numerous clinical trials that back the health benefits of beet roots. One such study published in the online journal of American Heart Association *'Hypertension'* discovered beets lowered blood pressure within 24 hours of drinking beet root juice[1, 2]. This is good news for people with high blood pressure as it provides a natural way to control blood pressure and perhaps one day limit the use of medicines.

In a separate study, it was found that the betacyanin in beet roots slows the growth of breast and prostate tumours by over 12 percent[3]. This is great news because the slowdown of cancer translates into more time for treatment of the cancer before it gets to the fatal stage.

Drinking beet root juice enhances stamina to exercise up to 16% longer. A University of Exeter study found that the nitrates in beet root juice reduce the oxygen intake, thus making exercise less tiresome. This level of reduction in oxygen intake cannot be attained by any other known means. Other than athletes, this finding can benefit the elderly and those suffering from metabolic, respiration, and cardiovascular diseases[4].

Resources:

[1]http://www.qmul.ac.uk/media/news/items/smd/31048.html

[2]http://www.nutritionj.com/content/11/1/106

[3]http://www.ncbi.nlm.nih.gov/pubmed/21434853

[4]http://sshs.exeter.ac.uk/news/research/title_37371_en.html

Blackberries

Introduction to Blackberries

The blackberry (also called bramble, brummel, brambleberry and bly) is an accumulation of numerous tiny fruits known as drupes. However, botanically speaking blackberries are not true berries. They are an aggregate fruit where each collection of drupelets develops from a single flower and each cluster is consumed whole and not as single units. The blackberry is a deep purple colored fruit, with fragile smooth skin. The centre of the fruit holds a greenish core that penetrates to the bottom of the fruit. It belongs to the Rosaceae family which is a wide ranging group with more than 375 species.

Blackberries are natural inhabitants of a number of continents. The domesticated varieties of the plant have been used as borders for property protection, for medical uses and human consumption. Due to the fruit's fragile nature and short shelf life, almost 90% of blackberries are used in frozen form. Classification of blackberries is determined by the type of the plant. There are the upright, semi-straight and trailing varieties of plants which are further divided into thorny and thorn-less cultivars. The semi-straight and trailing varieties of plants require extensive framework for support while the upright plants require no such support. The plants can reach as tall as ten feet and the fruit can be harvested from stems that are two years old. Properly maintained plants can produce fruit for as long as fifteen years.

History of Blackberries

The exact origin of blackberries is difficult to trace, the blackberry plant is a native of North and South America, Africa, and Australia. It is the most geographically spread fruit known. Greeks and Romans employed blackberries in medicines and the Native Americans used them as dyes, medicine and for food. In some cultures they were believed to offer protection against curses and spells provided they were collected during specific phases of the moon. It was also believed that boils were cured by crawling through blackberry bushes. Ancient Greeks depended on the blackberry to cure gout; this influence was so strong that in the eighteenth century they were commonly known as 'goutberry'.

Initially blackberries were not cultivated and simply grew in the wild. Anyone wanting the fruit would have to find bush growing in the wild and gather the berries. In Europe, blackberries have been used for more than two thousand years. Germans called blackberries 'brombeere' while in old English they were known as 'bramble'. Ancient Anglo-Saxons used the fruit to bake primitive pies in celebration of the first fruit feast of Lughnasadh at the start of August. In ancient times the blackberry was not used too frequently, but its roots, leaf and bark were employed for medicinal applications. They were used to treat whooping cough, venomous bites, boils and sore throat. According to some documentation they were even used to cure ulcers in 1771.

Health Benefits of Blackberries

The phytochemicals, minerals, vitamins and fibre work collectively to lower the danger of heart disorders, according to the publication of an article in "Nutrition Reviews" in 2010. This is carried out by minimizing inflammation and oxidative stress when antioxidant concentration is increased in the blood through the consumption of blackberries. The Anthocyanins in berries are responsible for the dark colour of the berries, combined with the elelagic acid they also make potent antioxidants that are believed to provide protection against cancer and chronic disease.

Regular use of blackberries may also help to prolong age related cognitive function. According to a study published in a 2009 issue of "Nutritional Neuroscience" animals fed with a 2% blackberry enhanced diet, produced better results on short-term memory tests[1].

The elevated content of tannin in blackberries helps to not only cut down on inflammation but provide relief from haemorrhoids and alleviate diarrhoea. The large helping of vitamin K helps to clot blood and strengthen bones. It also helps to reduce the effects of nausea and vomiting in pregnant women. Phytoestrogens aid in soothing the symptoms of premenstrual syndrome. It is also believed that phytoestrogens may contribute to brain functioning and immune health. Salicylate, a substance most commonly found in aspirin and pectin aids in lowering of cholesterol. Vitamin C is another overwhelming antioxidant that improves the immune system. Blackberries also protect the skin against premature wrinkles and other age related damage.

Nutritional Value of Blackberries

According to some sources blackberries top more than one thousand antioxidant foods in U.S.A. A one cup serving of blackberries provides 32% of the fibre requirement for the day at 8 grams. Additionally it delivers one gram of fat, two grams of protein, 14 grams of carbohydrates and only 62 calories. It is a mighty provider of vitamin C, supplying fifty percent of the daily requirement. Vitamin C is crucial in cell repair, fighting against free radicals and repairing wounds. It supplies 36% of the daily needs of vitamin K, which is needed for blood clotting. Furthermore, it delivers 9% of the folate requirement, which is essential in preventing neural tube birth defects, creation of DNA and red blood cells. One cup also provided 7% of a day's needs of magnesium and potassium, 6% needs of vitamin A and E, 5% of iron, zinc and niacin.

Blackberries are also rich in many phytochemicals like polyphenols, flavonoids, salicylic acid, ellagic acid, tennins, gallic acid and anthocyanins. Blackberries also have many big seeds which are not always favored by customers, but they too contain important nutrients. They house oils loaded with omega-3 (alpha-linolenic acid) and omega-6 fats (linoleic acid), along with carotenoids, ellagic acid, ellagitannins, dietary fibre and protein.

Blackberries consumed soon after harvest have the highest nutritional benefits. However, according to some evaluations frozen blackberries do not lose any significant amounts of nutrients. As a matter of fact, some sectors believe that if a fruit is allowed to ripen properly on the bush, and frozen immediately they might be better than those that sit on store shelves or ripen during transport.

Uses of Blackberries

All parts of the blackberry plant have been used throughout history. Indigenous America Indians used blackberry vines to make twine, while they were planted around European villages for protection against large wild animals. The berries were used to make the Indigo coloured dye. Beyond the practical uses of the tree itself, the berries have long since been turned into pies, crumbles, jams and more recently as flavouring for frozen yoghurt, ice-creams, and smoothes.

One of the easiest and best ways to use blackberries is to juice the berries for a refreshing nutrient loaded drink. For the sweetest, and best tasting juice pick the ripest berries that are firm and not over done. Berries not fully ripe will yield juice that is sour while overripe berries may contain parasites. After a through wash in cold water, follow the instructions for juicing.

Sweet Blackberry Juice

- Pulp the berries by hand, or in a blender.
- Allow the pulped berries to stand for half an hour. This allows the juice extracted to settle and draws additional juice from the flesh.
- Strain the rested juice then press the remaining pulp through a strainer while lightly pressing with the back of a spoon or a spatula. This will allow the maximum juice to be drawn out. For individuals wishing to retain more pulp in their juice strain through a coarse colander and for those who enjoy their fruit without any pulp, cheesecloth might be a better option.

If you pick your own berries during peak season, the juice can be extracted and frozen for several months in a sealable container. Otherwise, it can be kept in the refrigerator for a couple of weeks.

To make topping for pancakes, waffles or even ice cream the juice can be thickened. Use one cup of sugar for each one cup of blackberry juice (may be adjusted to personal tastes), and boil down to desired thickness.

Clinical Trials

It appears that adding more blackberries to your diet may help to lower the risk of cancer. According to a "Journal of Agriculture and Food Chemistry" study published in December 2006 blackberry extracts hindered the growth of cancer cells. The greater the quantity of extracts, the greater the amount of blocking that took place. The extracts were tested on human oral, breast, prostate, and colon tumor cells[2]. The nutrients responsible for this blocking include flavonols, anthocyanins, gallotannins, proanthocyanidins, flavanols, ellagitannins, and phenolic acids.

The German agency for regulating herbs, Commission E, has permitted the use of blackberry leaf tea for diarrhea. It is believed the tannins in the leaves are responsible for the ease of the problem. The commission recommends 4.5 grams daily as the standard dose. The University of Maryland Medical Center recommends one piled teaspoon of dried leaves for each cup of water to be consumed every half an hour[3]. Blackberry leaves have also been approved for treating mild inflammation of the mucous membranes, meaning that drinking blackberry tea can be beneficial for sore throat, gum inflammation and sores in the mouth.

Resources

[1]http://www.ingentaconnect.com/content/maney/nns/2009/00000012/00000003/art00005

[2]http://www.ncbi.nlm.nih.gov/pubmed/17147415

[3]http://www.livestrong.com/article/257328-what-are-the-benefits-of-blackberry-leaves/

Blueberries

A member of the Ericaceae family of the genus Vaccinium, the blueberry plant is a deciduous shrub. It exists as three different varieties known as highbush (Vaccinium corymbosum), rabbiteye (Vaccinium ashei), and southern highbush (Vaccinium formosum), and each variety thrives in different conditions and areas. The Highbush normally does well in cold climates and self-pollinates, but the size of the fruit and yield is better with cross pollination. The Rabbiteye prefers the warmer climate of southern United States, and does not self-pollinate. It requires two different plants for pollination. The Southern Highbush is a cross between the other two. It too self-pollinates but size and yield is better when there is cross pollination.

Blueberries have long been accredited with longevity and wellbeing. Recent studies indicate that when compared to all other vegetables and fruits, blueberries offer the maximum antioxidants for health protection. These elements are known to inhibit cell damage that can lead to cancer, in addition to minimizing age related diseases.

History

Native to North America, blueberry plants mostly grew in the wild along the eastern seaboard, starting as far north as Canada and extending all the way down to Florida in the south. The bilberry is a close cousin that is frequently mistaken for blueberries, as are 'huckleberries'. One way to distinguish them is by colour. Blueberries are always blue, while huckleberries and bilberries are generally red or purple.

Blueberries were mainly consumed by the Native American tribes and not very popular with the newcomers. The Hopi knew them as 'moqui' roughly meaning spirits of the ancestors. The native tribes dried the berries for use in puddings or even smoked them to use during the winter months when food was scarce. An amalgamation of fat, buffalo meat, and berries known as Pemmican, was used by the Native Americans for barter with companies trading in fur. A diet of Pemmican provided excellent nutrition with protein from the buffalo meat, energy form the fat, and vitamins from the berries.

Blueberries gained popularity during the American Civil War, where canning started so that they could be dispatched to Union Soldiers. With the start of their cultivation in the twentieth century, blueberries became a major industry in Canada and the United States.

Nutritional Value

Blueberries are a powerhouse of nutrients. Abound with vitamins A, C, E, and K, minerals potassium, iron, magnesium, and manganese, and phyto-nutrients Carotene-ß and Lutein-zeaxanthin. They are high in fibre and contain almost no saturated fats or cholesterol.

The large variety of antioxidants found in blueberries gives them many of the health benefits the berries are famous for. The Anthocyanins in the blueberries provide them with their characteristic blue colour which is water soluble. This turns the mouth, contact with skin, and fabrics blue upon contact. These antioxidants are found commonly in the plant kingdom, but blueberries have the highest concentration. Another antioxidant found in blueberries is Chlorogenic acid. It is believed to help fight free radicals and decrease the speed with which glucose is released into the bloodstream. Ellagic acid is thought to attach to cancer causing chemicals making them ineffective. Blueberries also contain plenty of catechins, the very same phyto-chemical that makes green tea a star. The antioxidant properties of catechins are believed to prevent plaque formation in arteries. Pterostilbene is still another antioxidant that is believed to help fight cancer and bring high cholesterol down. Finally there is Resveratrol. It offers a number of health benefits like anti-cancer, aging, plus inflammatory benefits along with life extending, and neuro-protective advantages. All this makes blueberries one of the best foods one can enjoy.

How to Use Blueberries

While blueberries make a tantalizing addition to pancakes, muffins and cheesecakes, by far the best way to fully benefit from their nutritional value is to consume them fresh. This can be done in the following ways:

- Combine fresh blueberries with yogurt for a nutritious breakfast or snack that provides plenty of protein, calcium, fibre, and vitamins. This will surely give you a great energy boost.
- Add a cup full of fresh blueberries to breakfast cereal. Not only will this contribute to a well-balanced diet, but it will also give you with a great start to any day.
- Blueberries can be eaten on their own, or they can be added to granola or trail mix for a delicious snack.

Blueberries are naturally very sweet tasting and can even cover the flavour of some veggies that may be added to smoothies. Being dark coloured, blueberries usually turn smoothies into very appealing purple shades. These qualities make them ideal for combining with other products to create great tasting drinks. The blueberry & yoghurt rave recipe below is an example of one such treat.

Blueberry & Yogurt Rave Recipe Ingredients:

1 cup of blueberries

1 cup of blueberry yogurt

1 teaspoon of honey

1/2 cup of ice

Directions:

Place ice, honey and yogurt in a blender and blend for 30 seconds at medium speed. Add the blueberries and blend for another 30 seconds. That's all there is to it.

Clinical Trials

A large number of independent clinical studies are being carried out on blueberries to fully understand their benefits. A study published by the Harvard School of Public Health, found consuming three or more servings of blueberries each week cut down heart attack risk in women by 33%. Researchers credited this to the high content of anthocyanin in the berries, which keep the arteries dilated to counter plaque accumulation[1].

In another study on the effects of blueberries and cognitive regression, Elizabeth Devore of Brigham & Women's Hospital and Harvard Medical School, found that consuming blueberries on a regular basis helped to reduce cognitive weakening. The trial made use of over 16,000 women from one of the largest studies in the US on women's health. The study concluded that eating as little as one serving of blueberries a week helped regress cognitive decline by many years[2].

According to a study headed by Dr. Rui Hai Liu (a Professor in the Department of Food Science at Cornell University in Ithaca, NY.), it was determined that antioxidant activity of blueberries was better than two dozen other fruits tested. Among those fruits were pomegranates, cranberries, red grapes, strawberries and apples. Antioxidants are linked with cancer prevention, anti-aging and heart benefits[3].

A number of studies relate the consumption of blueberries to cancer prevention. An especially difficult to treat form of breast cancer called Triple Negative Breast Cancer, was found to be inhibited with the use of blueberries by scientists at the Beckman Research Institute of City of Hope, California, U.S.A.[4] In another study carried out at the University of Illinois, Urbana-Champaign, by Mary Ann Lila, Ph.D., found that constituents in blueberries may be valuable in inhibiting different stages of cancer[5].

Intestinal bacteria play a positive role in our digestive and immune health. Researchers from Universities of Milan and Maine, headed by Dr. Stefano Vendrame, found through clinical trials that regularly consuming blueberry drinks favourably promoted the 'good' bacteria 'Bifidobacteria[6].

Resources:

[1]Aedin Cassidy, Kenneth J. Mukamal, Lydia Liu, Mary Franz, A Heather Eliassen, Eric B. Rimm. Circulation: Journal of the American Heart Association 2013; 127: 188-196

[2]Devore E E, KangJH, Breteler MM, Grodstein F. Annals of Neurology. April 2012: doi: 10.1002/ana.23594.[Epub ahead of print]

[3]Wolfe K L, Liu RH. Journal of Agricultural and Food Chemistry. 2008; 56(18): 8418-8426

[4]Adams LS, Kanaya N, Phung S, Liu Z, Chen S. The Journal of Nutrition, August 31,2011; doi:10.3945/jn.111.140178

[5]Schmidt BM, Howell AB, McEniry B, Knight CT, Seigler D, Erdman JW Jr, Lila MA Journal of Agricultural and Food Chemistry. 2004; 52(21): 6433-6442.

[6] Vendrame S, Guglielmetti S, Riso P, Arioli S, Klimis-Zacas D, Porrini M. Journal of Food Science. 2000; 65(2)

Broccoli

Brassica oleracea italica, or more commonly referred to as broccoli, is a native of the Mediterranean. Ancient Etruscans, considered the horticultural geniuses of their time, engineered broccoli from a relative of the cabbage plant. It is basically a large flower that can be eaten. Both the stalks and florets can be consumed raw or cooked. The leaves tend to be bitter tasting and therefore usually discarded, but some chefs can prepare them in specialised ways. Broccoli is a relative of cauliflower, and Brussels sprouts.

Cultivation of broccoli started in Italy and was given the name of Broccolo, meaning "cabbage sprout". The name derived from "brachium", a Latin word meaning arm or branch, an indication to its tree-like structure of a thick stalk divided into smaller stems, and ending in a thick head of florets. It is also sometimes known by its Italian name Calabrese, named in recognition of the Italian province Calabria where it was first cultivated. There are many varieties of broccoli ranging in colour from dark green to purple-green and even deep sage.

Broccoli is particularly loved by the Americans, according to the statistics put out by the National Agricultural Statistics Service, USDA. The average American consumes over four pounds of the vegetable each year. The USA is the third largest broccoli producer in the world, with more than 90% of the vegetable being grown in the state of California. One of America's founding fathers, Thomas Jefferson, was also a big admirer of broccoli. He especially imported seeds from Italy to plant in his home at Monticello, Virginia as early as 1767.

Broccoli also has a close association with the James Bond Films. The Italian born American, Albert R Broccoli, was responsible for putting the Ian Fleming books on film. All of the James Bond movies made during his lifetime were produced by Mr Broccoli himself.

History

Normally, the Etruscan people are associated with Italy. However, they were initially known as the Rasenna and migrated from what is now Turkey (formerly Asia Minor). It was here, in the region of Rasenna, that the cultivation of cabbages (predecessor to broccoli) was started by them. In the eighth century BCE, the Rasenna migration to Italy started and the knowledge travelled with them. The mobile trading of the Rasenna, with Phoenicians, Sicilians, Greeks, Corsicans and Sardinians, eventually led them to Rome, where some of them settled in the area of Tuscany. These immigrants were called "Tusci" or "Etrusci" by the Romans, and ancient Tuscany was referred to as Etruria.

An Italian naturalist and writer (23 – 79 CE) named Pliny, records that Romans cultivated broccoli in the first century CE. Initially, Romans enjoyed the purple sprouting variety that took on a green colour when being cooked. Later, a variety called Calabrese was developed, and it is the most commonly used type even today in the United States. Broccoli has been considered to be a precious food by the Italians ever since the Roman Empire. In fact, it was initially introduced into the USA by Italian immigrants.

Health Benefits

Broccoli is a superhero of the veggie kingdom. This is due to the health benefits that are associated with the plant. The high levels of potassium not only aid in optimal functioning of the human brain, but also keep the nervous system healthy and enhance the growth of muscles. The large quantity of soluble fibre in the vegetable is good at eliminating cholesterol from the body. Additionally, this same fibre also helps to keep a check on digestive issues and constipation, while giving the feeling of being fuller for longer periods of time, thus contributing to maintaining healthier levels of blood glucose.

Dr. Peter Hoagland and Dr. Philip Pfeffey, of the U.S Department of Agriculture, found in their research that broccoli contains the fibre called calcium pectate. Calcium pectate attaches to bile acids thereby keeping more cholesterol in the liver and allowing less into the blood. They learned that broccoli is just as efficient at lowering cholesterol as some cholesterol medicines.[1] The chromium found in broccoli may be useful at preventing the onset of diabetes in some adults. Dr. Richard Anderson of the US Department of Agriculture (an expert in diabetes) found chromium to boost insulin's ability to function better.[1]

Broccoli is also credited with detoxifying the body because of the beta carotenes, vitamin C, calcium phytochemicals, and the indoles and disothiocynates found within it. These enzymes further help to prevent heart disease, osteoporosis, and cancer, in particular prostate, cervical and breast cancers. The Magnesium, calcium, and potassium found in broccoli, are thought to help regulate blood pressure.

Broccoli also contains certain components that can be harmful if caution is not practiced. For individuals on blood thinning medications, excessive amounts of broccoli is not advisable. This is because it may impede with the functioning of those medications and increase the risk of stroke. Consuming more than two cups of broccoli in one day may also enhance the chances of developing kidney stones.

Nutritional Value

Proper preparation of a vegetable is important in retaining the maximum nutritional value it has to offer. To get the best flavour and nutritional value out of broccoli, it is best to use it soon after purchase. Even when refrigerated a vegetable loses its flavour and a considerable amount of the vitamin value over time. Cooking veggies also impacts their ability to provide the right amounts of nutrients. For attaining the greatest nutritional value out of broccoli, it is best eaten raw.

After five minutes of boiling, broccoli loses 20 - 30% of its cancer fighting compounds like sulforaphane. Ten minutes of boiling and this goes up to 40 - 50%, and thirty minutes takes away as much as 77% of the anti-carcinogenic properties. Other cooking methods, like microwaving, steaming, or stir frying, do not have any substantial effect. Broccoli has an abundance of vitamins, and minerals. It contains vitamin B1, B2, B3, B6, C, iron, Folic acid, magnesium, potassium and zinc. The dark green colour of the vegetable indicates its rich content of vitamin A.

One cup of cooked broccoli provides 71.8 mg of calcium, which is what one would get by drinking 4 oz. of milk. The same one cup delivers 116.4 mg of vitamin C, a quantity contained in one whole orange. This fulfils the daily adult requirement of vitamin C. One cup also provides 10% of the daily iron needs, while the vitamin C helps in the absorption of the iron. Additionally, it delivers 4 grams of protein yet only 44 calories. This combination of beneficial nutrients makes broccoli the ideal diet food. Usually, frozen broccoli contains roughly 35% more beta carotene compared to the fresh kind. This is simply due to the fact that most of this substance is found in the florets, and frozen packages are mostly florets. However, the stems contain extra calcium, iron, thiamin, riboflavin, niacin and vitamin C. Putting it simply, the whole broccoli flower should be consumed to get the full benefit of all its nutrients.

How to Use

Wash broccoli with cold water and divide the florets into quarters so they cook evenly. Trim away and discard any woody parts of the stem and any hard leaves. Peel the remaining stem and cut into ½ inch slices. To gain all the unique health benefits, make sure you let the cut broccoli stand for several minutes before cooking.

To attain the maximum nourishment, cook broccoli in a temperature range of 212°F (100°C), with a cooking time of no more than five minutes. Since the stems are fibrous and take longer, they should be cooked apart for a few minutes, prior to adding the florets.

The best way to cook broccoli is to steam it. Just fill the bottom of a steamer with two inches of water and allow it to boil. Put the stems in first, and after two minutes add the florets for a maximum of five minutes. Remove and top with optional ingredients as desired, things like cheese, yoghurt, or a Mediterranean Dressing. Steaming preserves the flavonoids, B complex vitamins, and vitamin C, as well as carotenoids and glucosinolates in the vegetable.

Stir-frying broccoli is another cooking option. However, there is the risk of nutrient damage from the high oil heat. To stir fry broccoli, heat the pan to 248°-284°F (120°-140°C), for no longer than three to three and a half minutes. When cooked in this way, roughly two-thirds of the nutrients are retained. To retain greater nutritional value, the heat can be maintained at the lower end (approximately 250°F/121°C), and the frying time reduced to three minutes. This will help to retain more than two-thirds of the nutritional value.

Clinical Trials

[1] Studies carried out by Nutrilite Health Institute to determine the effects cooking had on the beneficial compounds in broccoli, found that the glycosinolates in the plant are transformed into isothiocyanates (ITCs), which are associated with powerful antioxidant properties. Within a few hours of eating either fresh or steamed broccoli, ITCs were found in the blood of participating volunteers.[2]

Research carried out at Linus Pauling Institute at Oregon State University, discovered that the "sulforaphane" found in broccoli provides not one, but two ways to prevent cancer. While the actual studies were carried out to research the compounds effect on prostate cancer, researchers say the effect will most probably be the same on colon and breast cancers[3].

A laboratory study funded by Arthritis Research UK, the Biotechnology and Biological Sciences Research Council's (BBSRC) Diet, Health Research Industry Club (DRINC), and The Dunhill Medical Trust, found that sulforaphane in broccoli slowed down the damage to human cartilage in joints. Researchers claim that a diet rich in this compound can help with diseases like osteroarthritis[4].

Resources

http://www.vegparadise.com/highestperch44.html

[2]http://www.nutrilite.com/en-us/Science/NHI/BestOfScience/broccoli.aspx

[3]Oregon State University (2012, February 28). Eat your broccoli: Another mechanism discovered by which sulforaphane prevents cancer. (http://www.sciencedaily.com/releases/2012/02/120228140555.htm)

[4]http://www.uea.ac.uk/mac/comm/media/press/2013/August/broccoli-osteoarthritis-research-sulforaphane

Brussels Sprouts

Introduction to Brussels Sprouts

Botanically brussel sprouts, scientific name *Brassica oleracea* (variety gemmifera), belong to the Brassica family. This family contains a large number of vegetables we eat, including cabbage, horseradish, broccoli, turnips, mustard, cauliflower and kale to name a few.

The sprouts are actually leaves that have been customized. The clusters of leaves superimpose over each other tightly and give a ball like shape, with the net result of green buds looking like minute cabbages. Rows of sprouts develop along each long stem of the plant. Initially they start as bumps at the base of the stalk and move upwards. To get sprouts that are of uniform structure, it is customary to cut off the tip of the stalk as soon as sprouts begin developing at the stalk bottom. The size of the vegetable varies from half an inch to two inches in diameter. The plant has a fairly long growing season with the fall harvest being more abundant and flavorful.

History of Brussels Sprouts

Brussels sprouts have been cultivated for over 2,500 years, growing during the winter months and providing highly nutritive food during the colder winters of thousands of years ago. It is believed that the original vegetable that *Brassica oleracea* belongs to, grew wild along the Atlantic seaboard of Europe and the Mediterranean basin. Many different types of vegetables have been developed through selective breeding of advantageous characteristics. These include collard, with extra large leaves, kale with curled leaves, cabbage the terminal bud, Brussels sprouts with large leaves folded into a tight mass and kohlrabi with enlarged stems. Broccoli and cauliflower are actually overly grown flowers.

While the Brussels sprouts cultivar's (specifically bred rather than wild) is not known exactly, the French are credited with coining the term in the 18th century. During those times it was common to put a landmark label on the food, regardless of whether they were developed in Brussels, Belgium or not.

There is documentation of Brussels sprouts in the location of present day Brussels dating as far back as 13th century, hence the name.

Brussels sprouts continued to exist as a local crop until their spread throughout Europe during World War I. They were initially introduced to America in the 1800s by the French. Today nearly the entire Brussels sprout crop grown in the U.S is from California and nearly all of it ends up as frozen products. As luck would have it, despite the fact that the roots of Brussels sprouts lie in Belgium, it is the Netherlands that are Europe's key producer of the vegetable.

Health Benefits of Brussels Sprouts

Brussels sprouts are a hugely nutritious vegetable that offer protection against a large number of modern day ailments. When steam boiled, they provide some unique cholesterol-reducing benefits. The fibrous components found in the veggie bind better with bile acids in the digestive tract when cooked in this way. This makes it easier to remove them from the body with the net result that cholesterol is lowered.

Brussels sprouts have an exclusive ability of protecting DNA. Upon regular consumption of the vegetable, certain constituents in the sprouts block sulphotransferase enzymes. This in turn improves the stability of DNA in white blood cells. Brussels sprouts are a rich source of glucosinolates, important phytonutrients known to be the chemical initiators of many cancer-protective materials. For example the glucoside, sinigrin destroys pre-cancerous cells in the colon. The Zea-xanthin is an important carotenoid absorbed by selection into the eyes, where it provides light-filtering duties of UV rays and prevent retinal destruction as well as age related macular degeneration in the elderly. Additionally, Brussels sprouts supply these nutrients, unlike some other cruciferous vegetables, without endangering the thyroid gland.

The Di-indolyl-methane in Brussels sprouts is a successful anti-bacterial and anti-viral substance. Together the antioxidant vitamins C, A and E eliminate the body of harmful free radicals. Vitamin K plays an important role in maintaining bone health and aid in minimizing neuron damage which delays the onset of Alzheimer's.

Consumption of Brussels sprouts also delivers a number of important minerals. Potassium is needed in cells and body fluids to control heart rate and blood pressure, manganese is a co-factor needed for antioxidant enzyme superoxide dismutase while iron is needed for cellular oxidation and generation of red blood cells.

Nutritional Value of Brussels Sprouts

Brussels sprouts have many good points. To start with they are low in calories and sodium, totally free from cholesterol and very high in dietary fibre. In the mineral department they are very high in manganese and potassium and high in iron, magnesium and phosphorus. In the vitamin department they are very high in vitamins A, B6, C and thiamin, and high in riboflavin. They also provide some thiamine, folate, niacin and riboflavin. Finally, Brussels sprouts are rich in a number of important phytonutrients.

A one hundred gram serving of the veggie provides only 43 calories, and 15% of the daily recommended allowance of fibre, 15% vitamin A, 142% vitamin C, 4% vitamin E, 221% vitamin K, 15% folate, 11% vitamin B6, 9% thiamin. Brussels sprouts are a potent source of some vital minerals. They supply 8% of the daily iron needs, 11% of potassium, 7% phosphorus, 6% magnesium, and 17% manganese.

Uses of Brussels Sprouts

Brussels sprouts are a traditional winter food in UK, usually consumed boiled especially at Christmas time. However, there are numerous other ways of using them. They may be oven roasted, stir-fried, steamed or made into a soup.

To prepare the sprouts they should be washed and the base with any portion of stem removed. Next remove any leaves that become lose due to the cutting of the base and discard. A lot of people cut a cross into the stem when boiling or steaming to speed up the cooking process by allowing the penetration of heat to the middle of the veggie, but I prefer to cut the sprout in half. Excessive cooking the sprouts can lead to the release of sulfur compounds in the vegetable, which makes them release an unpleasant odour reminiscent of school dinners. Blanching the sprouts in boiling water for five minutes and cooling before addition to recipes will eliminate this problem.

Quick Serving Ideas

- Microwaving and lightly topping with butter and seasoning with herbs.
- Roasting and salting. A favorite snack in Europe.
- Blanching and combining with other vegetables like green beans, mushrooms or carrots.
- Use as a side dish with roasts or chicken casseroles.

Roasting Technique

After preparing according to the above instructions, place the sprouts in a large bowl. Lightly drizzle with olive oil and sprinkle to taste with coarse salt, and freshly ground pepper. Thoroughly toss the sprouts so all of them are properly coated. Layer them individually on a cookie sheet and allow them to roast in an oven preheated at 425°F (220°C) for approximately 20 minutes. When half cooked, the sprouts should be turned once and then allowed to finish cooking.

Sprouts in Salad

Steam Brussels sprouts and put aside (you can put them in ice water to help preserve shape and colour, and stop them from over-cooking in their own heat). In a bowl slice red onions, toss in mild cheese of choice (feta or goat cheese are good), walnuts and the sprouts. Add balsamic vinegar and olive oil and toss to allow all flavors to blend. Enjoy as a side dish or on its own as a great tasting salad.

Clinical Trials

The Beta-carotene, sulforaphane, indole-3-carbinol, 3,3'- diindolylmethane and a number of other glucosinolates in Brussels sprouts have been found to suppress the progression of cancer in human breast cells[3]. Furthermore they have exhibited the effect of chemotherapy drug Taxol, while the kaempferol in the sprouts might offer protection against cardiotoxicity[1, 2].

A number of clinical studies have shown Brussels sprouts to be beneficial in conditions like gastric ulcers, cardiac conditions, asthma, morning sickness and *Helicobacter pylori* infection. In addition it is believed that sprouts may help against conditions like macular degeneration, lung, stomach and prostate cancer. The sprouts also show some promise as antacids, and mild laxatives. Being anti-bacterial, anti-fungal, and anti-viral, the sprouts are also beneficial against many skin disorders. Lastly applications of brassica leaf extracts have helped relieve swelling in lactating women.

Resources

[1]http://foodforbreastcancer.com/foods/brussels-sprouts

[2]http://lpi.oregonstate.edu/infocenter/phytochemicals/isothio/

[3] http://www.naturalnews.com/029204_broccoli_cancer_cells.html

http://naturalstandard.com/index-abstract.asp?create-abstract=brassica.asp&title=Cabbage,%20Broccoli,%20Cauliflower,%20Collard,%20Kale,%20Brussels%20sprouts,%20Kohlrabi

Cabbage

Introduction to Cabbage

Brassica olerocea, more commonly referred to as cabbage is a member of the Brassica family just like cauliflower, Brussel sprouts and kale. Cabbage is composed of a gathering of stiff leaves overlying on top of each other in compact layers, leading to the net result of a globular shape. There are a number of varieties cultivated around the world the main ones of which include green, red and savoy. The group is divided into two basic categories early and late. The early variety attains maturity in a little over forty days and has a smaller, tight head while the late variant takes almost ninety days to fully develop.

The green variety ranges in colours from a pale shade of green to dark green. The red variant has leaves that maybe range from purple to crimson shades with numerous white veins running through the leaves. The leaves of both varieties are smooth-textured, while the Savoy cabbage has leaves that are more ruffled. Its taste too is milder, not as crunchy textured as that of the red or green varieties. The leaves closer to the centre are usually paler in colour than those found on the exterior as they are protected from the sunlight.

Cabbage grows well in cooler climates and yields hefty harvests. It also stores well when not in season; this is why it is a favoured food. The added benefit of the vegetable is that it is very nutritious and offers significant medicinal value. The English name of "cabbage" is most probably derived from the Picard dialect of Old French word "caboche", which means head.

History of Cabbage

Pots holding cabbages dating as far back as 4,000 B.C.E. have been discovered in the Shensi province of China. It is believed that origins of cabbage lie in north China, where the ancient people thought of it as a 'cooling' food in the yin and yang concept. While cabbage is frequently associated with the Irish, the Celts are accredited with carrying it from Asia to Europe around 600 B.C.E.

Cabbage plays a role in Greek mythology too. It is an agriculture fact, and also known to the Greeks that grape vines do not flourish if grown near cabbage. According to one Greek myth Dionysus, God of wine wandered into Thrace followed by his loyal companions the Bacchae. The land of Thrace was under the control of Lycurgus and threatened by the arrival of the newcomers, Dionysus and his companions were captured. To avenge his capture, and being a God, Dionysus had Lycurgus driven mad. Not being in the right frame of mind, Lycurgus thought his son was a grape vine and proceeded to hack it to pieces. Realizing what he had done, he wept and the tears falling to the ground from his eyes sprang up as cabbage.

The ancient Romans too loved their cabbage. Cato recommended consumption of vinegar soaked cabbage before excessive use of alcohol. The standard remedy in Roman times for a hangover was ingestion of cabbage. In addition to being a food source for Caesar's armies, wounded soldiers were bound with cabbage leaves to help reduce infection. The conquering Romans introduced Cabbage into Europe where selective cultivation led to the cabbage we are familiar with today. In Europe cabbage caught on fast and became a popular food item, partly due to the good nutritive contributions it made to the scanty diet of the rural population.

Cabbage was one of the food items carried on ships of explorers during the seventeenth and eighteenth centuries due to its good storage qualities and high vitamin C content that helped to keep scurvy, a common ailment among sailors of the time, at bay. According to history, the sailors injured in a storm during one of Captain Cook's voyages were bound with cabbage to help avert gangrene.

Health Benefits of Cabbage

Fresh cabbage leaves are not only highly nutritious but provide a large variety of health benefits. Its high vitamin K content plays a critical part in clotting of blood and maintenance of bone strength. Lack of this nutrient can lead to early development of osteoporosis or uncontrollable bleeding if injured. Vitamin K also has a vital job in curing Alzheimer's disease by minimizing neuronal damage in brains of patients suffering from the disease.

Each cup of cooked cabbage delivers four grams of dietary fibre, which contains both soluble and insoluble fibre. Consumption of soluble fibre is related lowering the risk of diabetes and high cholesterol while insoluble fibre aids in the regulation of bowel movements. Cabbage has been called one of the best overall sources of dietary fibre and ingestion of fibre-rich foods might aid in the prevention of heart disease, obsesity, cancer, hemorhoids, and constipation.

One cup of raw, shredded cabbage delivers approximately 30% of the recommended daily allowance of vitamin C. This important vitamin prevents free radicals in the body from damaging healthy cells and supports healthy blood vessels, and skin. It further reduces chances of cancer, hypertension, and heart disease.

Like other members of its family, cabbage houses an elevated concentration of glucosinolate compounds. When chewed thoroughly and digested these compounds decompose into indole and isothiocyanates. According to the National Cancer institute these compounds are strong antioxidants that have the potential of averting the growth and migration of tumour cells by killing prospective cancer causing cells.

Phyto-chemicals such as like *thiocyanates, lutein, indole-3-carbinol, sulforaphane, zea-xanthin, and isothiocyanate are also found in cabbage.* These compounds are strong antioxidants known to offer good protection against colon, breast and prostate cancers. Furthermore, they help to bring down the levels of LDL "bad cholesterol".

Cabbage also contains sufficient amounts of vital minerals like manganese, iron, potassium and magnesium. Potassium helps to control blood pressure and heart rates while iron is needed for the formation of red blood cells. Manganese is a co- factor for antioxidant enzyme and iron is necessary for the formation of red blood cells.

Nutritional Value of Cabbage

Cabbage is the perfect food for people trying to lose weight. A hundred gram serving delivers only 25 calories, contains no cholesterol or fats of any kind and hardly any sodium. The same one hundred grams offers 6%, (based on a 2,000 calorie diet) of the daily recommended carbohydrate needs, 2.5% of the dietary fibre, 1.3% protein.

It is also a rich source of an array of vitamins and minerals delivering 72% of the daily vitamin K in a single 100 gram serving, 44% vitamin C, 11% vitamin B-9 (folate), 10% vitamin B-6, 5% vitamin B-1, 4% vitamin B-5, 3% vitamin B-2 (riboflavin), and 2% vitamin B-2.

In the mineral department the one hundred gram serving supplies 8% manganese, 4% phosphorus, calcium, iron, and potassium, 3% magnesium, 2% zinc and 1% sodium.

Cabbage leaves also contains glutamine, the substance responsible for its anti-inflammatory properties. Different varieties of cabbage also contain different amounts of glucosinolates which can be converted into isothiocyanate compounds that fight a number of cancers including bladder, breast colon and prostate.

Uses of Cabbage

Proper preparation of cabbage is essential for getting full nutritional value it has to offer. The vitamin C decomposes quickly if exposed to light, water, air and heat. Cabbage should be cut just before eating and it best when stored in a cool dark place. Also use the vegetable within three to four days of purchase. The enzyme myrosinase in cabbage converts glucosinolates to cancer preventing isothiocyanates. Seven minutes of steaming breaks down as much of the myrosinase as two minutes of mirowaving. Hence, short steaming is better than microwaving to attain full value of the veggie.

The slightly bitter flavour of cabbage is actually a good thing. One of the glucosinolates responsible for the taste, called sinigring is found in high quantities in cabbage. It too provides the anti-cancer properties cabbage is known for, and while food industry tries to remove this taste through hybridization, it is best to keep it and blend cabbage with foods that will mask the bitterness.

To allow the anti-cancer myrosinase enzymes do their job, you need to slice, shred, or chop the raw vegetable and allow it to stand for five to ten minutes before steaming it. When the cells are broken through the cutting process, the myrosinase enzymes need the time to become active for the process of converting glucosinolates to isothiocyanates.

Cabbage is enjoyed around the world in a variety of ways. Sauerkraut and coleslaw are forms of salad enjoyed all over Europe, while in Ireland they enjoy it as colcannon. Hungarians stuff cabbage and Koreans prepare kimchi. Raw chopped cabbage leaves can be added to any salad preparations. It can also be made into a soup like preparation with beet juice or added to yogurt to prepare "borscht" so popular in eastern European countries.

Clinical Trials

The complex phytonutrient compounds found in cabbage make it one of the best natural treatments for ulcers. In a study carried out at San Quentin Prison in California, 93 percent of the patients with duodenal ulcers were healed after just three weeks of cabbage juice consumption. They were given the equivalent of one quart of fresh cabbage juice daily[1].

According to research conducted by the U.S Department of Agriculture, red cabbage houses 36 varieties of anthocyanins, types of flavonoids that have been linked to averting cancer. A Japanese study found that anthocyanins amend the way fat cells function and might help in fighting metabolic syndrome. Metabolic syndrome is a group of symptoms associated with diabetes, cardiovascular disease, and high blood pressure[2].

Resources

[1]http://www.naturalnews.com/027454_cabbage_ulcers.html

[2]http://www.naturalnews.com/024487_cabbage_red_cabbage_anthocyanins.html

Cantaloupes

Introduction to Cantaloupes

Cantaloupe is a fleshy fruit with strong musk like smell and sweet taste. The skin has a dry, coarse texture. The scientific name for cantaloupe is *Cucumis melo* and it is a member of the same family as cucumbers, squash, pumpkin and gourds, growing on long training vines. Initially, there was only one true cantaloupe, the kind grown in Europe, but more recently the word cantaloupe has come to mean all melons having orange flesh. The European variety (*Cucumis melo cantalupensis*) or the true cantaloupe is recognized by its greenish-orange flesh, smooth skin, and prominent ribs similar to those found on a basketball. The North American variety (*Cucumis melo* var. *reticulus*) is really a muskmelon, sometimes referred to as rock melon due to its rock-like look and netted rind.

The true cantaloupe was cultivated in America until the late 19th century, but the easier to grow and more sun loving netted variety with longer growing season became more popular. Eventually only the latter variety was cultivated commercially but the name cantaloupe stuck.

History of Cantaloupes

Cantaloupes are believed by some historians, to initially have been cultivated in Greece and Egypt during the biblical times as long ago as 2400 B.C. Historical evidence points to extensive cultivation of melons in the region of the Nile valley. Some Egyptian paintings even have depictions of melons. Others claim that their origin lies in Iran, Armenia, and India. The Romans used melons in cooking as indicated by "Apicius", a book of Roman recipes, and it is believed that they got their supplies from Armenia. The initial fruits were much smaller that the varieties common today, and probably not as sweet either.

Serious cultivation of cantaloupes started in Italy in the fourteenth century. Through selective breeding, the Italians improved the size, quality and taste of melons. It is believed that the name "cantaloupe" developed from the town in which they were first cultivated after having the seeds brought over from

Armenia. According to legend, they were cultivated in the Papal gardens in the town of Cantalupo, near Tivoli. The only issue is that there were around seven towns with this name in Italy at the time and even one in France. So it is difficult to say with any precision where they were cultivated first, other than that they were cultivated in that region.

Due to the work done on cantaloupes by the Italians, the popularity of the fruit grew and spread into Spain during the fifteenth century. The Arabs established the trade of cantaloupes through their settlements in Andalusia. Christopher Columbus transported the seeds to the Americas on his second voyage and introduced them to the various locations he sailed through including Jamaica, Cuba, Hispaniola and Puerto Rico. France started cultivating cantaloupes in the seventeenth century, and referred to them as "sucrins" meaning sugar. Today cantaloupes are cultivated on all continents of the planet other than Antarctica.

Health Benefits of Cantaloupes

Cantaloupes are prized for their sweet taste, enticing aroma, and low calorie content. One cup of diced melon has only about 60 calories and is 89% water. It is the perfect addition to any summer diet to help keep you hydrated. They are jam packed with nutrients that provide a truck load of health benefits.

Cantaloupes contain large amounts of beta-carotene, which is converted by the body to vitamin A. Both of these are essential for good eyesight. High amounts of vitamin A consumption can reduce the incidence of cataracts by as much as 40%, thus reducing the risk of cataracts surgery. Additionally vitamin A helps to eliminate dry eyes, improve night vision and reduce macular degeneration of the eyes. One cup of diced cantaloupe provides a day's supply of this nutrient.

The potassium in cantaloupes is essential for contraction of the heart and a number of other smooth muscles in the body. It regulates heartbeat thus promoting oxygen supply to the brain and regulating the amount of water supply in the body. As a result you feel more relaxed and stress free. Potassium also helps to excrete sodium from the body and is beneficial for people with salt-sensitive hypertension. While excess amounts of potassium can be toxic for individuals with kidney problems; acquiring too much of the mineral by consuming cantaloupes is unlikely. Cantaloupes also contain a micronutrient myoinositol, a lipid that helps with anxiety and insomnia. They also have the largest amounts of digestive enzymes.

The nutrients and minerals combined in cantaloupes equip the body to recover from nicotine withdrawal. For someone trying to stop smoking, the regular use of cantaloupes in the diet will make the process easier. Also smoking exhausts the vitamin A in the body, and intake of cantaloupe will replenish it with beta-carotene.

Another compound found in cantaloupes is adenosine. This is usually given to heart patients as it has blood thinning abilities. Thin blood means there are fewer chances of clots hence, fewer chances of strokes of heart-attacks. Folate is another compound present in the fruit which is important in keeping the cardiovascular system healthy.

A glass of cantaloupe juice is beneficial for women near the time of menstruation. It helps to reduce excessive flow and clots while minimizing muscular cramps due to potassium deficiency. It is also a valuable source of vitamin C, an antioxidant responsible for removing cell damaging, free radicals from the body and strengthening the immune system.

Nutritional Value

Cantaloupes are great because one cup of the diced fruit delivers no fat, no cholesterol and only around 60 calories. It also provides fibre, protein and host of other micronutrients, vitamins and minerals. The same serving delivers 120% of the recommended daily value of Vitamin a, 108% of vitamin C. It satisfies 2% of the daily needs of each of the following calcium, iron, riboflavin, pantothenic acid and zinc. It also supplies 3% phosphorous, 4% copper, 5% magnesium and thiamin, 6% niacin and vitamin B6 and 14% potassium.

Uses of Cantaloupes

Cantaloupes are not suitable for cooking, but they can be used raw in fresh sweet and savory preparations. Cantaloupes can be enjoyed as breakfast fruit or in salads and as a part of cold desserts. In salads they combine well with feta and goat cheeses, almonds, hazelnuts, citrus and mint. They are ideally suited for turning into smoothies and juices.

Spiced Cantaloupe Smoothie - Makes two servings
Ingredients:

- 10 ice cubes
- 1 cup cantaloupe
- 3 0z. plain yoghurt
- 1½ Tbsp sugar, or if you prefer use honey instead
- ¾ fresh ginger grated

Add everything in a blender and puree until smooth. Sugar or ginger can be adjusted according to taste.

Another great way to enjoy cantaloupes is to make melon-lollies. This is a summer treat even the kids can't pass up.

Melon Lollies

Ingredients:

- 4 cups cantaloupe, diced
- 1 lime
- 1 Tbsp. honey (optional)

Directions:

- Blend the juice of one lime with the diced cantaloupe in a blender, and blend for 30 seconds.
- Pour the mixture into molds and freeze for a minimum of eight hours.

For the melons which have been left out and become overripe with soft spots, simply juice them. A melon that might not be the optimal texture for eating is perfect for juicing. Just cut and throw out any parts that appear to have external mildew. Cut it up and juice it with seeds and all. Research carried out at the University of Innsbruck, Austria, indicates that fully ripe fruits, even to the point of spoiling contain more antioxidants than under-ripe fruits. A major point to note is that a lot of the cantaloupe's nutrients are housed in the rind. So when juicing, cut close to the outer netted skin, keeping the maximum amount of the green inner layer, and juice it with the rest of the melon.

Clinical Trials

Cantaloupes work well as beauty products too. The beta-carotene, when converted to vitamin A in the body helps to produce clear fresh looking skin. It thins the exterior layer of skin containing the dead cells which can clog pores and even lead to blemishes[1, 2]. Another benefit of cantaloupes is that they help to prevent wrinkles. According to studies, beta-carotene helps to enhance skin elasticity and stop skin's premature aging[3].

The American Cancer Society advocates the use of melons as potent components in the battle against intestinal cancer and the more common melanoma (skin cancer).

Resources

[1]Does the plasma level of vitamins A and E affect acne condition? El-Akawi, Z., Abdel-Latif, N., Abdul-Razzak, K. Department of Biochemistry and Molecular Biology, Jordan University of Science and Technology, School of Medicine, Irbid, Jordan. Clinical and Experimental Dermatology, 2006 May;31(3):430-4.

[2]Vitamin a: history, current uses, and controversies. Chapman, M.S. Section of Dermatology, Department of Surgery, Dartmouth-Hitchcock Medical Center, Lebanon, NH. Seminars in Cutaneous Medicine and Surgery, 2012 Mar;31(1)11-6.

[4]Differential effects of low-dose and high-dose beta-carotene supplementation on the signs of photoaging and type 1 procollagen gene expression in human skin in vivo. Cho, S., Lee, D.H., Won, C.H., et al. Department of Dermatology, Seoul National University Boramae Hospital, Seoul, Korea. Dermatology, 2010;221(2):160-71.

Carrots

Introduction to Carrots

Carrots are a biennial plant from the parsley family initially grown for its scented leaves and seeds and not the roots. A few of carrot's relatives still cultivated for their leaves include funnel, dill, and parsley. Wild carrots belong to the *Daucus carota, Carota* sub-species while the domesticated carrots are members of Daucus carota, sativus sub-species. Wild carrots used to be red, white, black, purple but not orange! The best carrots for consumption are the slender, young ones. While baby carrots are appealing, they are not as flavourful as fully grown ones due to their lack of maturity.

When worn by the ladies of the English court, the lacy green foliage of carrot tops made an appealing hair, or hat ornament and was taken as a fashion statement. The ancient Greeks used carrots to prepare a love potion that was believed to endow men with passion while making women more submissive. The Romans believed the seeds and carrots to be aphrodisiacs and were a common sight in Roman gardens.

The root and leaves of the vegetable was used as yellow dye during the 16th and 17th centuries in Europe, and in France they are still used to make butter a little brighter in colour. Approximately one third of all the carrots dispersed in the world are produced in China, the largest producer of carrots in the world. Russia and United States closely follow China in world production of carrots.

History of Carrots

History of carrot extends back five thousand years. According to excavated evidence it is believed that they originated in Afghanistan. Travellers through the centuries dispersed the seeds along the trade routes of Africa, Arabia and Asia selling them in areas wishing to cultivate new and productive plants. The Greeks referred to the carrot as *Philon* or *Philtron* from their word *philo* meaning loving. Carrot's present name is inspired from the French who called it *carotte*.

The earliest varieties were more commonly used for medicinal purposes and less frequently as food. They were prescribed for a wide array of illnesses from treating syphilis to animal bites. King of Pontius (approximately 100 B.C), Mithridates, possessed a formula for neutralizing some poisons using carrot seeds as the main ingredient. Strangely enough the concoction has actually been found to work!

The early varieties were not very sweet or succulent like the ones today. European cultivation of carrots started in the Middle Ages with the Dutch developing the bright orange carrot by cross-breeding the red varieties with yellow – a colour inspired by the colour of the emblem of the House of Orange. Generations of selective breading finally produced the sweeter tasting succulent varieties most common today with a smaller inner core.

Health Benefits Carrots

Packed with an arsenal of nutrients, carrots are useful in fighting off a number of ailments. It is common knowledge that carrots are good for the eyes. This is because they are loaded with beta-carotene, something the liver converts into vitamin A and the retina transforms into rhodopsin, a purplish pigment needed for night vision. Beyond that beta-carotene protects against macular degeneration and old age cataracts and improves vision in general[1]. It is believed that consumption of beta-carotene can cut down on macular degeneration risk by as much as 40%. Additionally, it acts as an antioxidant countering cell damage due to routine metabolism. As such it aids in slowing down the aging process of cells.

Carrots contain falcarinol and falcarindiol which provide the veggie with anticancer properties. Falcarinol is a naturally occurring pesticide produced by the plant for protection of the root against fungal diseases. Carrots are just about the only ordinary sources of this compound, believed to be responsible for providing protection against lung, breast, and colon cancer[2].

The carotenoids beta-carotene, alpha-carotene and lutein are linked with lowering the risk of heart disease. Consumed regularly, the soluble fibres in carrots bind with bile acids to remove them from the body thus lowering the

LDL cholesterol. The potassium in carrots aids in improving blood pressure by lowering the effects of sodium[6].

Carrots house antiseptic and antibacterial properties that are ideal for improving the immune system. The high content of vitamin C fuels white blood cell (among the most relevant elements in human immune system) activity. Carrots act as potent antiseptics, helping to prevent infections when applied either as shredded raw, or boiled and mashed to external wounds.

Munching on raw carrots helps to scour off plaque like a toothbrush. Furthermore, carrots activate the production of saliva which is alkaline and counters the effects of acid and cavity forming bacteria. Eating raw carrots also stimulates the gums. The vitamin A nourishes the skin preventing dryness, blemishes and uneven skin tone.

Nutritional Value Carrots

The good thing about carrots is that they contain minute amounts of total and saturated fats, and no cholesterol making them a great diet food. They rate very low on the glycemic scale, getting 3 out of 100. This means that one serving of carrots has almost no effect on blood glucose levels, making it a good choice for diabetics.

The nutrients in carrots are packed in protein packets that need to be broken down to release the nutrients. So unlike most other vegetables where cooking cuts down the nutritional values grinding, cooking, juicing, or thoroughly chewing carrots only helps to release more of these nutrients. Cooking carrots in fats or oils, grinding, or juicing enhances the carotenoid availability by 600%. Carotenoids are fat soluble and presence of oils enhances their absorption by 1000%.

Just 100 grams of carrots provide 10 grams of carbohydrates, 1 gram protein and 3 grams fibre. The same quantity delivers roughly 10108 mcg beta carotene, 9.2 milligrams of vitamin C, 0.8 mg vitamin E, 0.147 mg vitamin B6, and 0.93 mg niacin. Additionally it contains vitamin K, thiamine, folate, and riboflavin.

Carrots also have ample amounts of minerals. In 100 grams of carrots there are 323 mg of potassium, 44 mg of phosphorus, 35 mg sodium, 27milligrams of calcium, 15mg magnesium, 0.6 mg of iron, 0.2 mg zinc and 1.1 mcg of selenium.

Uses

Besides tasting great when consumed raw as a snack, carrots can be eaten in many other ways. They can be boiled, steamed, sautéed, roasted, grilled, added to soups, stews, casseroles, quiches, omelets, stir fried and the list goes on. Their naturally sweet taste makes them a good ingredient in cakes, breads, muffins, or even cookies. Since, carrots can be used in so many ways, it only makes sense they should be purchased in bulk and preserved when in season to enjoy all year round. Here are some simple ways to do just that:

- Carrots keep for several months in the refrigerator.
- Dried carrots can be reconstituted for use in cooking. To dry fresh carrots simply wash young carrots and slice, shred or grate them. Add just enough lemon juice to lightly coat them and arrange on drying rack to dry to a crisp.
- Freezing carrots is very simple. After washing, cut them into desired sized pieces and steam until half cooked. Then submerge them immediately in cold water and store them in zip-lock bags.

Here are a few unconventional way to make use of carrots.

- To spike the nutritional value of soup. Replace cream or stock in creamed veggie soup with carrot juice. The juice makes a good enhancer and gives thick, pureed, root based soups more depth.
- Carrot juice can be blended into tomato based pasta or pizza sauces. Amount of juice used can be varied, replacing any portion or all of the liquid in the sauce. Blend some carrots in the juice and you have a great low fat topping for pasta, or seafood.

Chilled Carrot Milkshake
- 2 medium sized carrots
- 2 Tbsp honey

- Cinnamon, nutmeg, and allspice (a pinch of each)
- ½ cup plain yoghurt
- ½ cup milk

Method:

Wash and cut carrots into chunks. Steam until softened. Mash by hand or puree in a blender. Add all the ingredients and blend well. Chill before serving.

Clinical Trials

Carrots have shown promise in treating a number of ailments, among them, infantile diarrhoea. Two separate clinical studies indicate that carrots are beneficial for this condition. Other conditions in which carrots might be beneficial include vitamin A deficiency, constipation and antioxidant activity[3].

Anthocyanin is a forceful antioxidant in purple carrots. It provides natural protection against UV rays of the sun and aids in building collagen in the skin. In studies it has also shown promise in averting the growth of precancerous skin cells[4].

In a 2011 study, carrot juice extract was responsible for destroying leukaemia cells and prevent their progress[5].

Resources

[1]"Myth or Fact: Eating Carrots Improves Eyesight" DukeHealth.org. Accessed 13 December 2013.

[2]http://www.healthonlinezine.info/top-9-tips-to-prevent-breast-cancer.html

[3]http://www.naturalstandard.com/indexabstract.asp?createabstract=/monographs/herbssupplements/carrot.asp

[4]http://www.tauntongazette.com/health/x1146187974/The-skinny-on-skin-care

[5]*"Bioactive chemicals from carrot (Daucus carota) juice extracts for the treatment of leukemia."* Zaini R, Clench MR, Le Maitre CL. *J Med Food.* doi:

10.1089/jmf.2010.0284. 2011 Nov;14(11):1303-12. Abstract. Accessed 13 December 2013.

[6]http://www.sciencedirect.com/science/article/pii/S0944711300800641

Cauliflower

"A cauliflower is nothing but a cabbage with a college education." –*Mark Twain*

Introduction to Cauliflower

Regardless of the name, it is a vegetable and not a flower, belonging to the *Brassica Oleraces* species in the family of Brassicaceae. It is closely related to broccoli, cabbage, Brussels sprouts, and kale, which are also members of this species. Its name is derived from the Latin word *"caulis"* meaning cabbage with addition of *flower*. The name is in reference to the family known for producing only leafy greens for consumption.

The vegetable begins its development as a single condensed head, which is in reality an immature white flower bud, and reaches a size of seven to ten inches when fully developed. The head is also at times referred to as a "curd" due to the similarity in looks with the curds in lumpy milk. It has a mellow sweet, nutty taste, and almost all parts of the plant are edible. The stalks, green leaves and the head, but most people only use the heads. The dense leaves surrounding the head keep it enclosed and protect it from direct sunlight. The lack of light prevents green chlorophyll from developing so this keeps the head a pure white colour.

The vegetable is cultivated in all parts of the world with new varieties being developed constantly. While the most commonly used variety is white, purple and green cultivars are also available.

History of Cauliflower

Cauliflower is believed to have originated in Asia as a wild cabbage, but was actually bred first by Mediterranean farmers about 2500 years ago. It was known as "Syrian Cabbage" for the longest time due to being wide spread in Syria, Persia, and Egypt. The Egyptians were growing it around 400 B.C.E. and the Romans also grew it.

Arabs appreciated cauliflower for its food value and pleasant taste. As the Arab Empire expanded, the vegetable landed in Spain, where it immediately became popular. At roughly around the same time it was introduced to Cyprus by the Syrians, from where it spread into Europe. Until about the late 1500s, cultivation of cauliflower was limited to the Italian peninsula. It was introduced to France in the sixteenth century, where it was highly valued by the court of Louis XIV. It was also appreciated in Brittany. Menon, an 18th century food writer recommended serving cauliflower in a sauce made with veal, ham and cream as an addition to stew of sweetbreads and mushrooms.

The nutritious veggie made its way to North America in the 1600s, but commercial development did not start until around the 1920s. It has since grown to become a part of the staple diet all around the globe. In the period between 2001 – 2011 commercial sales dropped by 35% in the UK, so cultivators started the development of brightly coloured varieties to sell in mixed rainbow pickings' to revive interests.

Health Benefits of Cauliflower

Cauliflower is not one of the better studied cruciferous vegetables from a health viewpoint. However there are a number of studies linking cauliflower supplemented diets with prevention of cancer. In particular bladder, breast, colon, prostate and ovarian cancers are targeted by this vegetable. This cancer-fighting ability is due to cauliflower's nutrient content that supports three of the body's systems that have close relation with cancer development. The three systems are the detox system, antioxidant system and inflammatory system. Extensive imbalance in any one of these systems increases risks of cancer development. Problems with all three at the same time will only increase the chances of disease.

Cauliflower contains phytonutrients known as glucosinolates that trigger detoxification enzymes and standardize their activity. The three active glucosinolates found in cauliflower are glucobrassicin, glucoraphanin, and gluconasturtiian. Failing to provide the body with appropriate detox support and yet continuing the consumption of damaging substances due to existing life styles increases the incidence of cancer.

Vitamin C and manganese are two of the main antioxidants found in cauliflower. Cauliflower goes beyond the basics and contains additional antioxidants like beta-carotene, ferulic acid, beta-cryptoxanthing, caffeic acid, quercetin, rutin, cinnamic acid, and kaempferol. The combined antioxidant support reduces cell stress by cutting down on damage to the cells caused by harmful molecules. This in turn reduces risks of various cancers.

The glucobrassicin in cauliflower can also be converted to an isothiocyanate compound called indole-3-carbinol (I3C), which is an anti-inflammatory molecule working at the genetic level to eliminate the development of inflammation at its earliest stages. The vitamin K behaves as a direct controller of the body's inflammatory response. Inflammation increases risks of cancers and other chronic diseases like cardiovascular issues.

The fibre content in cauliflower supports the digestive system. Additionally the sulforaphane created from the glucosinolates found in cauliflower protect the stomach's lining by inhibiting the overgrowth of the *Helicobacter pylori* bacteria in the stomach and limiting its ability to adhere to the stomach's lining. Other potential benefits of cauliflower include keeping a check on diseases like Crohn's disease, rheumatoid arthritis, inflammatory bowel disease, obesity, insulin resistance, and ulcerative colitis.

Nutritional Value

In addition to having a high content of fibre and protein, cauliflower is low in fat. Just a hundred gram serving of raw cauliflower provides 1.9 grams of protein and 2 grams of dietary fibre. Based on a 2,000 calorie diet, that means you get 5 percent of the recommended daily allowance of fibre and 3 percent of the protein. This same quantity contains 5 grams of carbohydrates (1% of daily allowance), no cholesterol and only 25 calories.

Cauliflower is well endowed in the vitamin and mineral department as well. It contains vitamin C, K, folate, B-1, B-3, B-5, B-6, iron, calcium, magnesium, potassium, phosphorus, molybdenum, and manganese. The B vitamins are essential to the metabolism of carbohydrates, protein and fats, while the minerals play an important role for intracellular electrolyte balance, and as co-factors for antioxidant enzymes.

Uses of Cauliflower

Cauliflower can be used in a number of ways. To prepare the veggie turn it upside down after washing it thoroughly and remove the stem just at the base where the florets all come together. Proceed to separate the florets into roughly equal sized pieces, cutting when the need to maintain the equal size arises. Now the pieces may be served raw, or cooked as desired.

Rapid cooking of the vegetable cuts down on the odour causing sulphur compounds, maintains crispness, colour and minimizes the loss of nutrients. Over cooking allows nutrients to trickle into the cooking water and wasting them. Steaming and microwaving best preserve the nutrient content. Cauliflower can turn yellow in alkaline water. To prevent this, a tablespoon of lemon juice can be added to water. Also, cooking in an aluminium or iron pot can cause the vegetable to change colour as the molecules in the cauliflower react with the metal. An iron pot will give the cauliflower brown or bluish-green colour.

 A few ways to enjoy cauliflower include:

- In a salad or as slaw - similar to it cousin cabbage, cauliflower make great addition to salads. One example is to mix it with white beans and fennel and top with a dressing of choice.
- Roasted - Roast the cut up pieces of cauliflower in an oven by lightly brushing with olive oil and seasoning with herbs of choice until crisp. It compliments any main course or on its own as a mid-meal snack.
- Mashed - A great alternative to mashed potatoes. Just steam and mash with a little coconut milk for a semi-sweet dish or use plain milk and add seasoning and herbs according to taste.

Clinical Trials

According to some studies the sulforaphanes in cauliflower have been found to be effectual chemo-protective agents. They provide protection against development of tumours in the "post-initiation" stage. Initial studies indicate that cauliflowers may reduce the overall risk of cancer in particular colon and prostate[1].

Use of cauliflower extracts in studies have shown a noteworthy rise in scavenging activity of free radicals, and inhibition of lipid peroxidation. The antioxidant activity is proportionally related to the phenolic content[2]. Workers at Göteborg University, Sweden, found cauliflower to be among the vegetables with the greatest content of plant sterols. These compounds are known to lower the serum cholesterol. Thus a greater dietary consumption of cauliflower can produce a positive impact on health.

Resources

[1] Clarke JD, Dashwood RH, Ho E. Multi-targeted prevention of cancer by sulforaphane.Cancer Lett. 2008 May 24. SOURCE CDC.gov

[2] Llorach R et al, Valorization of cauliflower (Brassica oleracea L. var. botrytis) by-products as a source of antioxidant phenolics. J Agric Food Chem. 2003 Apr 9; 51(8):2181-7.

[3]Normén L, Johnsson M, Andersson H, van Gameren Y, Dutta P. Plant sterols in vegetables and fruits commonly consumed in Sweden. Eur J Nutr. 1999 Apr;38(2):84-9.

Celery

Introduction to Celery

The French word "celeri," is derived from its Greek version and in turn it gives rise to the English language word "celery". Celery is a biennial plant belonging to the same family as parsley, caraway, carrots and fennel. It typically grows in bundles of stalks that range from twelve to sixteen inches in height. While the whole plant is edible, stalks are the most commonly consumed portion of the vegetable. The root portion of one variety of celery is known as celeriac and is more flavourful than the stalks. Originally the plant was cultivated for medicinal purposes but now it has become a part of the daily intake for dieters and health food advocates.

Essentially there are two main varieties grown. The celeriac, scientific name *Apium graveolens* var. *Rapaceum* is also known as turnip-root, root celery, and knob celery, and is valued for its nutty taste. The second variety, *Apium graveolens* var. *Secalinum* resembles an overgrown parsley plant in looks and is valued for its long ribbed stalks. Other than raw consumption, celery is also employed in blended drink by health conscious individuals.

Celery stalks really come into the limelight when the idea to use them as garnish for Bloody Mary drinks was born in 1960. An unnamed famous celebrity supposedly ordered his Bloody Mary at the Ambassador East Hotel and got it without the swizzle stick, so he grabbed a celery stalk from the nearest relish tray and proceeded to stir his drink, thus making history. The vegetable is so famous that it is even mentioned in Homer's Odyssey as "selionon."

History of Celery

The Greeks considered celery to be a holy plant during their classical period. Winners of the Nemean Games were adorned with its leaves in the much the same way the winners of the Olympic Games wore bay leaves. The Nemean Games were held every other year beginning in 573 in the city by the same name in south of Greece.

It is believed that celery originated in the Mediterranean basin. However ancient documents mention celery, actually a plant similar to it being cultivated for medicinal use well before 850 B.C.E. Its medicinal characteristics were most probably due to the precarious oils found in all parts of the plant but more so in the seeds. The veggie was used to treat conditions like poor digestion, flu, colds, water retention, spleen ailments and different kinds or arthritis and liver issues. Despite having origins in the Mediterranean region, the plant's wild relations were found growing in British Isles, Sweden, Egypt, Algeria, China, India, New Zealand, and southern parts of South America.

According to Roman tradition, celery was linked to bringing bad fortune under some circumstance, but it was still valued more for cooking than religious purposes. They actually used a wild form of celery for seasoning known as 'smallage.' In the seventeenth century the Italians started to domesticate the plant. After years of selective breeding they developed the sweeter tasting celery stalk we are familiar with today.

Health Benefits of Celery

Celery has a large number of natural macro and micronutrients making it an ideal health food. It is a very good detoxifying food. It acts as a diuretic, regulating the body's fluids. The potassium in celery adds to this benefit as some diuretics deplete potassium. Celery juice behaves as a natural tonic for dissolving and removing gall stones from the body, while regular consumption prevents their future formation. The natural fibre content releases nutrients that help to avert constipation and keep the digestive system in good health. A large number of detox diet plans recommend the addition of celery juice to the daily menu. It is also a natural appetite squelcher, making celery a good low fat food for people trying to lose weight.

Celery contains numerous compounds that prevent the spread of cancer. Acetylenics are known to stop the growth of tumour cells, while other compounds known as phenolic acids impede the action of the compounds called prostaglandins, which promote the growth of tumour cells. Coumarins are another type of phytonutrients found in celery that may help stop free-radicals damaging healthy cells and inhibit cancers of the stomach and colon. Vitamin C is an important antioxidant that further boosts the immune system.

Chinese medicine has recognized celery's ability to lower blood pressure. The phthalides in celery relax muscles surrounding the arteries, thus widening the blood vessels and allowing for unhindered flow of blood. The compound also lowers stress hormones, one of which causes the blood vessels to tighten. It is further believed that the compound butyl phthalide in celery plays a role in lowering LDL (bad) cholesterol. The ability of celery to increase the secretion of bile further helps to remove cholesterol from the body.

The polyacetylene contained in celery provides relief from all inflammation including rheumatoid arthritis, gout, bronchitis, osteoarthritis, and asthma. The phytonutrient luteolin obstructs the path of inflammation in the brain and also stops the excessive production of TNF-alpha, a compound directly responsible for inflammation. The elevated amounts of magnesium in the vegetable produce a calming effect thus allowing for restful sleep for insomniacs.

Celery might also aid in reducing sugar cravings. The vegetable is rated low in glycemic index, meaning that its carbohydrates break down gradually, allowing for slow release of sugar into the blood. This makes celery good for diabetics.

Nutritional Value Celery

A one cup serving of celery contains almost not fat or cholesterol and delivers approximately eighteen calories. It is a rich source of dietary fibre with one cup delivering 1.6 grams. According to some estimates, women need between 21 to 25 grams while men need 30 to 38 grams of fibre daily. It is also a good source of vitamin K. The recommended daily requirement of this nutrient is 90 micrograms and just one cup of chopped celery provides almost 30 micrograms. Vitamin K aids in promoting the health of the skeletal system in elderly individuals and plays an important role in blood clotting. It is also a good source of vitamin A with a single cup supplying 453 international units. Women need 2,333 and men need 3,000 international units daily. Vitamin A is important for normal reproduction as well as good eyesight, cellular communication, healthy heart, lung and kidney function.

A one cup serving also provides seven percent of the daily required amount of potassium, five percent of vitamin C and B6, four percent calcium and two percent magnesium. Additionally it supplies trace amounts of folate, molybdenum, manganese, vitamin B1 and B2, phosphorous, iron and protein.

Uses of Celery

The best way to enjoy celery is raw. However that does not mean it can't be used in numerous cooked dishes and in a variety of ways. Some interesting ways to enjoy celery include:

- Use chopped celery in salads or slice as sticks to use with dips, line the centre with nut butter and place sultanas at evenly spaced intervals to create "ants on a log" the kids will love.
- Stuff the centre of the stalks with low fat cheese and sprinkle with paprika to serve as appetizer.
- Prepare celery salsa by heating oil and adding a couple of cloves of finely chopped garlic, onion, tomato and celery. Pour tomato sauce into the mixture and allow it to boil until the celery and onion are tender. Add enough flour to thicken the sauce and season to taste. Serve with tortilla chips.
- Slice the celery at an angle about the length of your fingers and add it to stir fries. Celery retains its crunch even after quick cooking.
- Make creamy celery soup to warm you on cold days.
- Add celery to stews or casseroles to get more out of the vegetable.
- Use celery leaves as garnish or anywhere you might use parsley.

Celery juice is a good way to get all the benefits celery has to offer. Many people prefer to combine celery with other sweet juices to cut down on the saltiness that comes with the veggie. Celery, cucumber, carrots, and apples make good a combination.

Refreshing Veggie Combo
- 2 small carrots

- 2 small stalks of celery
- ½ beetroot (beet)
- ¼ teaspoon lemon juice
- ¼ teaspoon chopped ginger

Juice all ingredients for a drink that contains potent properties for maintaining cardiovascular health and fighting cancer. For a sweeter drink a little honey can be added.

Clinical Trials

Studies indicate that celery seeds might be valuable in treating dysmenorrhea, hypertension and act as mosquito repellent[1]. Celery contains a lot of sodium, however this is not the same as table salt. Typical table salt is made up of insoluble inorganic components which can lead to the formation of varicose veins, hardening of the arteries and a number of other problems. The sodium found in celery is organic and soluble. It is vital for the body, allowing it to process other nutrients absorbed by the body. All of the body's cells are covered in salt solution. Not maintaining the appropriate salt balance leads to dehydration. This is why celery is thought to be a good rehydrating drink[2].

According to a study carried out in Mainland China celery was found to reduce systolic and diastolic blood pressure. A significant difference in blood pressure was observed after taking a total of eight ounces in equal amounts of honey and celery juice three times a day[3].

Resources

[1]http://naturalstandard.com/index-abstract.asp?create-abstract=celery.asp&title=Celery

[2]http://www.naturalnews.com/024596_celery_blood_salt.html

[3]http://www.ncbi.nlm.nih.gov/pmc/articles/PMC3210006/#ref31

Cilantro & Coriander Seeds

Introduction to Cilantro & Coriander Seeds

Coriandrum sativum or cilantro belongs to the *Apiaceae* family and is a fast-developing, sweet-smelling herb that grows in cooler temperatures. Coriander actually describes the entire herbal plant inclusive of the stems, leaves, seeds and roots. In reality it is actually two treats in one, the leaves are known as cilantro (Chinese parsley) while the tiny seeds are normally called coriander. The entire plant is edible. The leaves give a musky, citrusy and some even claim it to be "soapy" flavour to Mexican, Thai and Chinese cooking. They are also used in Indian dishes and chutneys. The seeds deliver a taste of orange peel or lemony flavour and are used in traditional dishes in India.

The herb has gained more popularity recently due to all the health benefits it provides. The leaves including the stems are commonly used in salads, sandwiches or made into teas and juices. In Southeast Asia the roots are dug, chopped and used as additions to salty pickled condiments.

History of Cilantro & Coriander Seeds

Although not much is known about the origins of the coriander plant, it does have a very long history extending back many thousands of years. It is believed to be a native of the Mediterranean and portions of south-western Asia. Folklore claims to have it growing in the hanging gardens of Babylon to provide fragrance over 3,000 years ago, while experts believe it was used as far back as 5000 B.C.E.

Some shrunken mericarps (parts of the flower) have been found in the Nahal Hemel Cave in Israel and this is possibly the oldest coriander find. A small quantity of coriander mericarps have also been recovered from Tutankhamen's tomb, and since the plant does not grow in the wild in Egypt, it is assumed that it was purposefully cultivated by ancient Egyptians. It also appears that the herb has been cultivated in Greece since the second millennium B.C.E. A tablet discovered at the Pylos, refers to coriander being cultivated for production of perfumes. It seems as if the plant served dual purpose: the seeds were used as a spice, while the leaves for their flavour. There is also some archaeological evidence to back this up as large quantities of coriander were recovered from an Early Bronze Age site.

The Romans introduced coriander to northern Europe. A writer of the times, quotes in his works, a first century B.C.E. Roman writer suggesting "combining (coriander, seeds) with cumin and vinegar, rubbed into meat as a preservative". He also mentions that ancient Chinese believed the seeds to provide immortality, while it was used as love potion in the Middle Ages.

Coriander is also talked about in the Bible. When talking of God's gift to the children of Israel in the Book of Exodus, it says "it was like coriander seed, white." It is most likely that the Israelites learned of coriander in Egypt. The Roman writer Pliny also mentions that the best coriander came from there.

Coriander was written about by a British monk in the thirteenth century and mentioned in the oldest British piece on gardening in 1440. In the sixteenth century the herbalist William Turner claimed the seeds were useful in curing St. Anthony's fire, an agonizing skin disease. According to the writer Roy Genders, King James II of England had special honey water made with coriander seeds. He further states "[Coriander water] is a pleasing after-shave lotion and takes any inflammation from the skin."

Coriander plants were one of the first herbs to be grown by the American colonists in the New World. The French used distilled coriander to cook up a type of liquor. Now cilantro is cultivated in tropical as well as subtropical countries around the world.

Benefits of Cilantro & Coriander Seeds

Coriander has been used medicinally throughout history. It was used to provide relief from insomnia and anxiety in Iran, and has been employed as a diuretic in traditional Indian medicine. Now its benefits are understood better and recognized even more.

Being a good source of iron, phytonutrients and flavonoids, it protects the body against a number of ailments. Its juice aids in treating dysentery, indigestion, colitis and hepatitis. It lowers blood sugar levels, averts nausea and helps with digestion. When combined with a pinch of turmeric powder it becomes a remedy for pimples. Linalol is an oil in coriander that detoxifies the liver and builds appetite. It also acts as a blood thinner, thus preventing clots that can lead to strokes.

Boiled coriander seeds, consumed as a tea reduces menstrual flow and fluctuating mood swings. The plant has antibacterial, fungicidal and anthelmintic properties (expels parasitic worms from the body) which can be used to improve oral health, cut down on digestive spasms and eliminate abdominal pain. The antimicrobial compounds aid in curing small pox. One of its most recognized properties is its ability to fight off Salmonella, a bacteria with the potential to threaten life. The antifungal properties also help to treat dry skin, eczema and other skin ailments. Its heating, analgesic characteristics help in treating rheumatism and pain in bones. The seeds are a good source of fatty acids and proteic materials which are useful in bringing cholesterol levels down.

Cilantro is among the limited number of herbs employed for heavy metal detoxification. Drinking its juice can help detoxify you of metals like mercury, aluminium and lead to name a few. Removal of the heavy metals aids in prevention of Alzheimer's disease and memory loss. The plant also has a sedative and muscle relaxing effect.

Coriander is very good source of dietary fibre. Just a hundred grams of the seeds deliver 41.9 grams of fibre (with same amount of leaves delivering 2.9 grams). Most of this is in the form of insoluble fibre that helps to enhance bulk in the body and keep food moving through the digestive tract and ease constipation. One hundred grams of cilantro also contains a little over two grams of protein and 3.6 grams of carbohydrates.

Both the seeds and leaves are a good source of minerals like copper, iron, potassium, calcium, zinc, manganese and magnesium. The plant is also rich source of a number of vitamins like vitamin A, B6, C, E, K along with niacin, thiamin and riboflavin.

Additional compounds found in abundant amounts in the seeds include fatty acids like petroselinic acid, linoleic acid (omega 6), oleic acid, and palmitic acid. Essential oils found in the seeds include linalool (68%), a-pinene (10%), geraniol, camphene, and terpine. Fresh coriander leaves are a rich source of carotenoids. A 125 ml serving of fresh coriander leaf juice supplies nearly as much beta-caretene as 250 ml of broccoli juice.

Uses of Cilantro & Coriander Seeds

The popularity of cilantro and coriander seeds has increased tremendously in recent years. Some people claim they find the smell of fresh leaves distasteful, but they are in the minority. Those who are not bothered by the aroma consume cilantro leaves in salads, salsas, and layered onto all types of sandwiches. Cilantro is a vital topping of Thailand's favourite noodle dish. Additionally it can be used as a topping on rice pilaffs, spicy soups, beans and as an accent to chilli.

Coriander seeds can be roasted in a warm dry pan until you can smell the nutty fragrance. Roasting only takes a few minutes, but releases an amazing scent and essential oils. Once roasted, the seeds can be roughly ground with a mortar and pestle and used in a variety of dishes. Just a few seeds are sufficient for curry dishes, lentils, stews, mushrooms, rice, and any vegetable dishes of choice.

The leaves are a good addition to homemade pot-pourri. A few crushed seeds added to rose petals, lavender, or rosemary provide a subtle lingering perfume to any sitting room, office or bathroom. Oils from seeds are used in various commercial herbal medicines and as a flavouring in gin, vermouth, tobacco, and liqueurs.

Clinical Trials

According to some studies the antioxidants in coriander postpone and even prevent food from spoiling when it has been seasoned with the herb[1]. Both seeds and leaves contain antioxidants, but leaves have a more pronounced effect. Another study found that cilantro leaves are effective in fighting against Salmonella[2].

According to documentation coriander has been used to treat type 2 diabetes. A study using mice found that extract of coriander showed both insulin-releasing and insulin-type activity[3]. It has also been found that coriander seeds lower the total cholesterol and triglyceride levels. They increase the levels of high-density lipoprotein (good cholesterol). It is believed that this is due to liver increasing production of bile and speeding up of the breakdown of cholesterol into less harmful components[4].

Resources

1 Wangensteen, Helle; Samuelsen, Anne Berit; Malterud, Karl Egil (2004). "Antioxidant activity in extracts from coriander". Food Chemistry 88 (2): 293. doi:10.1016/j.foodchem.2004.01.047.

2Kubo, Isao; Fujita, Ken-Ichi; Kubo, Aya; Nihei, Ken-Ichi; Ogura, Tetsuya (2004). "Antibacterial Activity of Coriander Volatile Compounds againstSalmonella choleraesuis". Journal of Agricultural and Food Chemistry 52 (11): 3329-32. doi:10.1021/jf0354186. PMID 15161192.

3Gray, Alison M.; Flatt, Peter R. (2007). "Insulin-releasing and insulin-like activity of the traditional anti-diabetic plant Coriandrum sativum (coriander)". British Journal of Nutrition 81 (3): 203-9. doi:10.1017/S0007114599000392. PMID 10434846.

4Chithra, V.; Leelamma, S. (1997). "Hypolipidemic effect of coriander seeds (Coriandrum sativum): Mechanism of action". Plant Foods for Human Nutrition 51 (2): 167-72. doi:10.1023/A:1007975430328. PMID 9527351.

Cranberry

Introduction to Cranberry

Cranberry is a ruby-red coloured, tart berry that typically grows in the acid bogs. The plant is a low creeping evergreen shrub or vine that can measure up to two metres (7 ft.) in length and approximately five to twenty centimeters (2 - 8 inches) high. The slim, wire like stems are not overly woody and they hold the dark pink, refluxed flowers with exposed style and stamen. This allows for easy pollination by bees. The initially white fruit which develops is larger than the plant leaves, but turns a deep crimson colour when it reaches maturity. The acidity of the fruit overwhelms its sweet taste.

The botanical name for the most common type of berry is *Vaccinium oxycoccos*, or the European cranberry, a species native to Northern Europe, Asia and America. The name stems from the Latin word for cow *"vacca"* since cows seem to enjoy them too. The *Oxycoccos* is a reference to the plant's sharp leaves.

Cranberries are also referred to as "bounceberries" since they actually bounce if fresh ones are dropped and "craneberries" as poetic justice to their pink flowers which give the appearance of cranes that make the cranberry bogs their home. "Bearberries" is another one of their names because bears too love them. The commercially cultivated berries in the U.S and Canada botanically known as *Vaccinium macrocarpon,* are grown over stumpy trailing vines on top of sandy bogs. These yield larger sized fruit than those found in the wild and Europe.

History of Cranberry

The Native American Indian tribes were familiar with this multifaceted fruit and had their own names for it. The Lenni-lenape Indians of New Jersey, called it "ibimi" or "bitter berry", the Chippawas referred to it as "a'ni-bimin", the Alogonquin called it "atoqua" and Naragansetts named it "sasemineash". They used them as food and to symbolize friendship and peace. It was consumed raw or as a part of maple sugar mixture and even served with deer meat.

The Indians also recognized the preserving powers of the berries and frequently mixed them with pemmican (a mixture of dried meat) to preserve it. Additionally they were used for decorating purposes, to produce red dye and medicinally. The Indians made a wrap of crushed barriers to apply on wounds, where their astringent tannins helped to contract tissues and stop bleeding. We know that they also have antibiotic effects which probably helped to prevent infections as well.

The Pilgrims learned about the use of cranberries from the native tribes and were exporting them to England by the 18th century. In the days of the clipper ships, they were carried aboard in barrels to prevent scurvy. It is thought that cranberries were doled out in the early Thanksgiving dinners in Plymouth, Massachusetts. Cranberry juice was also extracted by the early settlers.

The resilient berries ended up in Holland by surviving a shipwreck. An American ship with crates of the fruit sank near the Dutch coast. A large number of the crates washed onto the island of Treschelling and took root. Cranberry cultivation has taken place there ever since.

Conscious cultivation of cranberries was initiated in 1840 when Henry Hall noticed that large sized berries began growing each time sand was deposited into his bog by prevailing winds and tides. The sand filled bog created the ideal conditions for growing berries by smothering the growth of low rooted weeds and promoting the growth of the deep rooted cranberries.

Health Benefits of Cranberry

The American Indians were always familiar with the medicinal properties of berries, but now even science collaborates this. Cranberries are not longer just a staple during the holiday season. The fact that cranberries treat urinary tract infections is a long established truth. Now we also know that they may enhance gastrointestinal and oral health, decrease LDL and elevate HDL (good) cholesterol, help to recover from stroke, and even provide help in preventing cancer. According to a study published in the "British Journal of Nutrition" in August 2006 and conducted at Laval University, Canada, a study group of obese patients registered an increase in HDL after consuming 8 ounces of cranberry juice daily for four weeks[1].

Vitamins C and E are antioxidants found in profuse amounts in cranberry juice, in addition to flavonoids that possess anti-inflammatory and anti-bacterial properties. Together they work to fight *E. coli*, bacteria that can cause urinary tract infection, eliminate *Helicobacter Pylori* bacteria from the body which is linked with ulcers and stomach cancer, and get rid of streptococcus mutants from the body, the bacteria known to cause tooth decay. The antioxidants also remove free radicals before they impair healthy body cells.

Consumption of cranberries is beneficial in preventing a number of cancers including breast, colon, lung and prostate. They are able to do this by blocking expression of MMPs (matrix metalloproteinases), inhibiting ODC (ornithine decarboxylase enzymes), stimulating QRs (quinone reductase enzymes) and activating apoptosis (programmed cell death) in tumor cells.

Nutritional Value of Cranberry

The fact that phytonutrients have cancer fighting capabilities is common knowledge, what may not be known is the fact that cranberries house a wide range of these powerful nutrients. Among them are phenolic acids like hydroxycinnamic, caffeic, coumaric, and ferulic acid, anthocyanins which include cyanidins, malvadins and peonidins, proanthocyanidins in particular epicatechins, flavonoids that include quercetin, myricetin, and kaempferol and the triterpenoid, ursolic acid.

Fresh cranberries are low in calories with a one hundred gram serving (approximately 1 cup) delivering only 46 calories. Same quantity also provides 12.2 grams of carbohydrates, 4.6 grams of fibre and 4 grams of sugar. In the mineral department as well they are not lacking with 7% of the Recommended Daily Allowance of copper and 20% of manganese. Noteworthy vitamins in a single serving include 13 milligrams of vitamin C which is close to 20% of the RDA, 6% pantothenic acid and 7% vitamin E.

Uses of Cranberries

While cranberries tend to be a bit too tart and many people prefer not to eat them out of hand, it does not meant they can't benefit from this valuable fruit. Cranberries can be wonderful additions to a large number of dishes starting with quick breads, salads, relishes, chutneys, salsas, moving on to soups, desserts, and entrees based on grains.

The tartness of cranberry can be used to replace the lemon or vinegar in a green salad. In a fruit salad they can be mellowed by combining with sweeter fruits like oranges, apples, pears or pineapples. Equal parts of cranberry juice and fruit juice of choice with sparkling mineral water produces a refreshing spritzer for a great pick-me-up. Add a handful of berries to a bowl of cereal for a perfect start to your day. Dried cranberries mixed with some salted nuts make a great midday snack.

A Few Quick Ways to Use Cranberries

- Throw in some dried cranberries to your favourite muffin recipe.
- Mix crushed cranberries, orange juice and honey to taste and freeze on popsicle sticks.
- In a food processor, puree cranberries with some orange juice and boil down to syrup-like texture. It creates the perfect complement on waffles or pancakes.
- Combine cranberry sauce and plain cream cheese for a great tasting bagel topping.
- When getting ready to bake apple, hollow out the core and stuff with cranberries mixed with sugar and cinnamon.

Clinical Trials

Urinary tract infection (UTI) is painful at best and cause permanent kidney damage in more serious forms. Women are prone to get it more frequently than men, with roughly half the female population getting some form of infection at some point in their lives. A randomized, placebo-controlled study conducted in Japan between 2007 and 2009 studied the effect of cranberry juice on patients with multiple relapses of the infection. The study subjects were patients aged between 20 to 79 years. The subjects were divided into two groups, with one group being given cranberry juice daily and the other a placebo drink. The patients drank 125 ml of the juice every night for twenty four weeks before going to bed. Recurrence of UTI was prevented in the group drinking cranberry juice[2, 3].

In a study carried out at the University Hospital in Olomouc, Czech Republic in 2010, the effectiveness of cranberry powder in men at risk of prostate disease with lower urinary tract symptoms was investigated. The evidence that cranberries may improve LUTS, a common ailment in older men was found, and as a result reduce the risk of prostate cancer.

According to a 2010 study carried out at William Harvy Rsearch Institute in England, cranberry juice cocktail daily can prove to be as good for the heart as red wine as both drinks promote healthy arteries. Tests were carried out using cranberry juice cocktail, light cranberry juice cocktail, a California merlot and an Argentine cabernet sauvignon on endothelin-1 (a marker of blood vessel dilation/constriction) and it was discovered that changes in both were similar[5].

Resources

[1]http://www.ncbi.nlm.nih.gov/pmc/articles/PMC3075541/

[2]http://www.ncbi.nlm.nih.gov/pubmed/22961092/Abstract

[3]http://www.sciencedaily.com/releases/2010/08/100823183807

[4]Vidlar A, Vostalova J, Ulrichova J, Student V, Stejskal D, Reichenbach R, Vrbkova J, Ruzicka F, Simanek V. The effectiveness of dried cranberries (Vaccinium macrocarpon)in men with lower urinary tract symptoms. British Journal of Nutrition 2010; 104:1181-1189.

[5]Caton PW, Pothecary MR, Lees DM, Khan NQ, Wood EG, Shoji T, Kanda T, Rull G, Corder R. Regulation of Vascular Endothelial Function by Procyanidin-Rich Foods and Beverages. Journal of Agricultural and Food Chemistry 2010; 58:4008-4013

Cucumber

Cucumis sativus, more commonly known as cucumber, is a member of the gourd (cucurbitaceae) family, which also includes gourds, melons and squashes. Another name for cucumbers is gherkins, which actually alludes to cucumbers in their pickled form. Currently, it is the world's fourth most commonly cultivated crop, after onions, tomatoes and cabbage. Even though we tend to think of cucumbers as vegetables, they are actually a fruit by definition. Fruits are produced by development of the ovary in the flowering plant.

Cucumbers can be divided into two main categories, those being pickled and those to be sold for eating raw. The pickling cucumbers are generally petite with thick, spiny dotted skins. Eating cucumbers tend to have smooth skin and are larger in size, with some varieties extending to over two feet long. While most people are accustomed to seeing green cucumbers, they actually exist in a wide array of colours and sizes. Cucumbers can be white, yellow, and even orange in colour.

The best known varieties of cucumbers existing today are a result of hybridisation carried out in the 1800s. Like all other members of this family, cucumbers are easy to grow and adapt to every growing zone with ease. They can be cultivated effortlessly on any upright supporting framework in the tiniest of gardens. The creeping vine grows up the frame and grabs them with skinny, spiralling tendrils. The large leaves hide the fruit under its canopy.

Cucumbers are loaded with vitamins, minerals, and phytonutrients, which make it a beneficial anti- inflammatory and antioxidant source. Since cucumbers are nearly 96% water, they are a great food for rehydrating in the long hot summers. Moreover, in some parts of the world they are sliced and sold on the streets and enjoyed fresh on sunny afternoons. The phrase "cool as a cucumber" is a reference to the cooling properties of the vegetable. The phrase was first documented to have been used in a poem entitled "A New Song" by the English poet John Gay in 1732.

History

Believed to be native to the foothills of the Himalayas, in an area that is now a part of India; cucumbers have been grown for around 4,000 years. Their use eventually spread into the Mediterranean and they were especially admired by the Romans, who eventually introduced them to Europe. The Roman Emperor, Tiberius, loved them so much that they were cultivated in greenhouses so that he could eat them all year round. Julius Caesar, another fan of cucumbers, enjoyed them most when pickled. Even Cleopatra accredited some of her beauty to cucumbers. Medicinally, they were used by the Romans to treat bad eyesight, scorpion bites, and to scare mice. Women wishing to bear children wore them on their waists.

The Spanish were responsible for taking them to the New World. Native-Americans started cultivation of cucumbers along with pumpkin and squash. Cucumbers gained such significance that they are even referred to twice in the Bible, in Numbers 11:5 and again in Isaiah 1:8. It is believed that the pickling of cucumbers started in the Tigris Valley around 3,000 years ago. Earliest forms of pickles were prepared by placing them in brine, later modifications were made and new spices added to create new versions.

In the 1600s, lots of people in England did not appreciate uncooked or fresh produce. This was due to the mindset that such vegetables were about as good as animal feed. As a result, cucumbers gained the unflattering nickname "cowcumber". Later, even as fresh vegetables started to become more popular, cucumbers remained ostracised for some time.

The flavour of cucumbers varies according to the sensitivity of one's taste buds. While the vast majority of people claim a watery like taste, or even a light melon-like flavour, a small minority say they have a very abhorrent taste. Sometimes, a few of the cucumbers growing on a plant can have a bitter taste, which is attributed to the chemical cucurbitacin. Cucurbitacin is generally poisonous to livestock, especially sheep.

Health Benefits of the Cucumber

Cucumbers are thought to be the perfect diet food because they have nominal calories and fat, and are loaded with nutrients. They are also used in beauty products like lotions, soaps, and facial masks. The ascorbic acid and caffeic acid found in cucumbers is responsible for lowering water retention which helps to reduce swelling and puffiness under the eyes. Cucumber skin provides relief to sun and wind burned skin.

Regular consumption of cucumbers is useful for aiding digestion. The dietary fibre along with high water content found in cucumbers is said to be responsible for eliminating toxins from the body, and also help with digestive disorders like gastritis, heartburn, ulcers, and even chronic constipation. The presence of silica helps to strengthen the connective tissues like tendons, cartilage and ligaments, and ease joint pain. Silica is also responsible for healthy nails. The photo-chemicals in cucumbers are good for eliminating bad breath. Simply place a slice of cucumber in the mouth for approximately thirty seconds, and then eat normally.

A combination of cucumber and carrot juice is accredited with lowering uric acid and helping to relieve gout and arthritis pain. Cucumbers also contain the hormone required by the pancreas to produce insulin, thus helping people suffering from diabetes, while the sterols in it help to lower cholesterol levels. The presence of potassium and magnesium in cucumbers help to regulate blood pressure, while the silicon and sulphur encourage hair growth. Just a 100 gram serving of cucumbers provides 150mg of potassium, which also helps to regulate metabolic rates and build muscle tissue. Potassium also enhances overall muscle flexibility.

The three lignans found in cucumbers are associated with reducing the risk of prostate, breast, and ovarian cancers. Due to the alkaline nature of cucumbers, drinking its juice is good for treatment of acidity and is good at calming gastric ulcers.

Nutritional Value

The whole cucumber is editable. The flesh contains vitamins A, C, and folic acid, and the skin provides fibre, and minerals like magnesium, molybdenum, and potassium. Additionally, the trace element silica, ascorbic, and caffeic acids, is also found in it. Other nutrients include vitamins B_1, B_2, B_3, B_5, and B_6, in addition to calcium, iron, phosphorus and zinc. The relatively high content of vitamin K in cucumbers is good for promoting bone mass.

The three different types of phytonutrients in cucumbers that are responsible for the antioxidant, anti-inflammatory, and anti-cancer activities, are Flavonoids, Lignans, and Triterpenes. In addition, this mix behaves as scavengers against the free radicals found in the body, which play a role in the aging process.

How to Use Cucumber

Cucumbers can be consumed raw, as additions to salads, or in a pickled form. Additionally they can be enjoyed as relishes, sauces in dressings, or as dill pickle. There are even a few ways to enjoy cucumbers by cooking them.

One particularly cool, creamy, and low-fat way of enjoying cucumbers, is to prepare them as a classic Indian side dish known as raita. This sauce goes well with lamb, sausage, rice, chicken, chops, and even fish. It may even be used as a dip for vegetables or with chips, and as a substitute for mayonnaise in a sandwich. Raita's creamy coolness offers a harmonious equilibrium with spicy foods.

Raita Recipe:

- 250 grams of plain yoghurt
- 1 Medium peeled cucumber, seeded, and finely chopped
- 10 mint leaves (approximately), also finely chopped
- ½ teaspoon of cumin seeds
- Salt and black pepper to taste

Directions:

Place the yoghurt in a deep dish and mix well so that it's creamy smooth. Add remaining ingredients, mix well and serve.

There are no hard and fast rules when it comes to making raita. To make is spicier, a finely chopped green chilly can be added. To make the raita runnier, just add a couple of tablespoons of milk. To further enhance its flavour, add a one or two finely chopped cloves of garlic.

Juicing cucumbers with skin, seeds, and flesh is a great way to get all the benefits from the many nutrients they have to offer. Cucumber's taste is so mild that it can be easily mixed with any other vegetable or fruit. Personally, I have found that cucumber juice can help mask the stronger flavours of other ingredients in the juice. Since cucumbers are mostly water, they yield a lot of juice. Just remember to wash it thoroughly before putting it in the juicer.

Cool Cucumber Concoction

- 1 large cucumber
- ½ peeled lemon
- 2 carrots
- 1 medium apple

Run all ingredients through a juicer and pour in a tall glass over ice.

Clinical Trials

Cucumbers have not been employed in too many studies or clinical trials. Most of the nutritional benefits of cucumbers are based on the detailed analysis of the nutrients found in them, and the studies of the health benefits that these individual nutrients provide. One particular study carried out in 2011 entitled "Clinical Sciences: Colours of Fruit and Vegetables and 10-Year Incidence of Stroke," did use cucumbers. In this study, fruits and vegetables were classified into separate groups based on the colour of their edible flesh. The vegetable colour reflects the quantity of advantageous phytochemicals like flavonoids and carotenoids present within them. Cucumbers fell into the white category along with apples and pears. The study found that orange/yellow, red/purple, and green fruits and vegetables, had no relation to incidence of strokes, while the frequency of strokes was 52% lower in people who consumed larger amounts of white fruits and vegetables.

Resources

http://www.examiner.com/article/can-apples-pears-cauliflower-and-cucumbers-help-reduce-the-risk-of-stroke

Dandelion Greens

Introduction to Dandelion Greens

What most people think of as a nuisance and a hideous weed is such a well respected plant that it sits on the U.S National Formulatory, as well as the Pharmcopeias of Poland, Hungary, Soviet Union and Switzerland. It is also one of the top six herbs in the Chinese herbal medicine. This is the common dandelion plant.

Dandelion plants are highly nutritious edible plants that are omnipresent and within easy access of everyone. The leaves are the more commonly consumed part of the plant however the root and flowers can also be eaten. While they may be consumed in raw form many people also cook them to tone down their bitter flavour.

Hundreds of varieties of the dandelion grow all over Europe, North America and Asia, in the more moderate climate zones. They are a hardy perennial plant that grows to roughly twelve inches in height when fully mature. The hairless, shiny leaves have jagged, toothy edges and are grooved to channel rain water into the roots. In fact the plants are known as "dent de lion" or "lion's teeth" in France, a reference to the long jagged leaves resembling a lion's mane. The stems of the plant are topped off with bright yellow flowers. The flowers open with the rising sun and close in the evening or during overcast weather. The brittle, brown roots are fleshy with milky white liquid. It is the liquid that gives the plant the bitter taste and a mild odour.

When harvesting your own leaves, it is best to pick from plants that have as yet not gone to flower. This is because the energy travels up to the flower, and as a result the greens become very bitter. Such leaves would require a number of blanching baths to cut down the bitterness. The flowers can be employed to make wine. Also avoid picking leaves from public places which might have been treated with insecticides and pesticides.

History of Dandelion Greens

Even though the dandelion had travelled significantly prior to written history, it can be stated with a fair degree of certainty that the plant is a native of Europe and Asia. Earliest recordings of the plant are seen in Roman times and its use is recorded by Normans of France and Anglo Saxon tribes of Britain. Arabian physicians were the first to note the use of dandelion for medicinal purposes in the tenth and eleventh centuries. The Welsh medicines mention it in the thirteenth century.

Dandelions have been intentionally carried throughout history across the lands and oceans by humans. The plants were carried to the New World by the Puritans because they were considered to be very useful. The primary planned reason for bringing dandelion to America was medicinal. Initially dandelions were not valued by the settlers as a food commodity. Another reason they cultivated it was because it was known to them and in an unknown land it reminded them of home.

Health Benefits of Dandelion Greens

Dandelion greens provide a large array of health benefits. Back in 1927 it was noticed that dandelions caused contraction of the gall bladder and promoted bile flow in dogs. Bile is a liquid produced by the liver and stored in the gall bladder until needed. Its job is to emulsify fats during the process of digestion. Use of dandelion enhances the flow of bile by three to four times. Dandelions can be used to treat inflammation of the bile duct, liver congestion and gall stones.

Japanese researchers in 1981 discovered that dandelions showed anti-tumour activity. There was clear correlation between timing of dandelion extract administration and the observed anti-tumour activity. It is believed that this activity is partially due to the nutritional content of the plant. Additionally dandelion has high content of the compound inulin, which is useful for diabetics in regulating blood sugar levels. High levels of blood sugar produce the damaging chemicals called glycation end products or AGEs that speed up aging, dementia, diabetes and cause cancer. The University of British Columbia reports in a 2004 study that dandelion flowers have high luteolin and luteolin-7-0-glucosid, both of which show major antioxidant and anti cancer benefits[1].

A 2007 study carried out by the Osaka City University Graduate School of Medicine in Japan discovered that dandelions heightened the activity of female hormone receptors in mice indicating that the herb might help reduce symptoms of PMS. According to the findings of the study, reproductive hormones act through receptors in body tissues and the more active the receptor become the greater the effect of hormones[2].

Nutritional Value Dandelion Greens

Dandelions rank in the first four positions according to USDA Bulletin #8, "Composition of Foods" (Haytowitz and Matthews 1984). While "Gardening for Better Nutrition" puts them in a tie for ninth place for all vegetables inclusive of grains, greens and seeds. The data further states that they are the richest green source of beta-carotene, precursor of vitamin A, and the third richest when considering all foods, following cod-liver oil, and beef liver. Dandelion is also especially rich in fibre, potassium, calcium, iron, phosphorus, magnesium. Additionally it is an excellent source of B vitamins, thiamine, riboflavin and protein. Russian and Eastern European studies by Gerasimova, Racz, Vogel, and Marei (Hobbs 1985) further indicate that dandelion is loaded with micronutrients like copper, zinc, cobalt, molybdenum, boron and Vitamin D1[3].

Other nutritional components found in dandelions include flavonoids, among them a number of luteolins that also act as antioxidants. The leaves contain natural chemicals called terpenes giving the leaves their bitter taste and plant sterols such as beta-sitosterol and stigmasterol. The plant sterols have a structure that resembles cholesterol. They provide natural anti-inflammatory properties and aid in cutting down on the absorption of dietary cholesterol into the blood stream.

Uses of Dandelion Greens

As a rule it is best to use dandelion greens as soon as they emerge out of the ground. The longer they are allowed to mature, the more bitter they become. They can be use raw to add a new layer of flavour to salads and in the same way as chicory or endive. Cook dandelion by lightly steaming or sauté with other vegetables. If they are too bitter, boil them by changing water several times to wash out the bitterness. The flowers can be steamed, fried or used in brewing wines. Flowers can also be eaten as pickled condiments. The roots may be boiled, roasted, or stir fried. Roots pair well with naturally sweet vegetables like carrots, or yams.

Not only can dandelion tea be therapeutic but it can be the perfect substitute for those trying to give up coffee. It provides the energy lift similar to that of coffee without the caffeine. Dandelion coffee for ready use is typically made by roasting and grinding dandelion roots. Once the powder is made, it can be used in water just like instant coffee. The powder is almost identical to real coffee and users claim it is better tasting than low quality coffee. Some people add dandelion powder to real coffee or chocolate to give it a better flavour.

Since dandelion greens tend to be bitter, it is a good idea to combine them with something sweet to cover the flavour. This is why they go great in a smoothie. Combining chopped dandelion greens with favourite fruits in season like mango, citrus, pineapple or strawberries not only taste great but provide a truckload of healthy nutrients.

Dandy Smoothie

- 1/2 cup water
- 1 cup chopped dandelion greens (loosely packed)
- 1 small banana
- ½ cup strawberries
- Honey or other sweetener of choice (if needed)

Directions

Place all ingredients, except sweetener and blend for approximately thirty seconds. If you prefer extra sweet then add desired amount of sweetener at the end.

Clinical Trials

Dandelion leaves are recommended as supplementary food for women who are pregnant due to the numerous nutrients they house. Additionally they have been shown to produce diuretic effect which makes them useful for PMS syndrome. Like other bitter herbs, dandelion root can be used to enhance appetite[4].

The University of Maryland Medical Centre states that foods containing high amounts of oxalates and calcium can lower the occurrence of kidney stones. Dandelion is naturally high in oxalates and when eaten in combination with foods high in calcium, the two compounds bind in the intestines thus protecting the kidneys[5]. Columbia University claims that dandelion leaves made into tea can reduce swelling and fluid retention in addition to promoting weight loss[5].

Resources

[1]http://www.amazing-green-tea.com/dandelion-health-benefits.html

[2] Zhi X, Honda K, Ozaki K, Misugi T, Sumi T, Ishiko O (2007). Dandelion T-1 extract up-regulates reproductive hormone receptor expression in mice. Int J Mol Med. 2007 Sep;20(3):287-92. - See more at: http://www.amazing-green-tea.com/dandelion-health-benefits.html#sthash.aVTh9pwK.dpuf

[3] http://www.leaflady.org/health_benefits_of_dandelions.htm

[4] http://www.med.nyu.edu/content?ChunkIID=21667#ref2

[5]http://www.naturalnews.com/040713_dandelion_edible_weeds_health_benefits.html

Fennel

Cultivated all over the globe now, Fennel (Foeniculum Vulgare) is originally a native of the Mediterranean. It belongs to the Umbellifereae family and is a close relative of dill, carrots, coriander and parsley. Fennel is a perennial herb that has a whitish, pale green bulb, with overlaying stalks extending out of it, which are similar to those found in celery. The hollow stalks end in feather like green leaves, close to where yellow coloured flowers grow producing the fennel seeds. The fennel plant can grow up to heights of three feet. All parts of the plant bulb, stalk, leaves, and seeds can be eaten, but it's usually the dried seeds that are used in cooking. The plant propagates rather easily and in many cases is thought to be an invasive group.

Consumed raw, fennel has a pleasant aroma and a crisp texture with a mildly sweet but assertive anise like flavour. Upon cooking the flavour mellows in comparison. The herb is especially associated with Mediterranean cuisine and in particular with Italian cooking. The seeds are commonly used in meatballs and sausages in Italy as well as rye breads in northern Europe. The bulbs can be consumed raw in salads or used in side dishes with pastas and risottos. A number of egg and fish dishes use dried and fresh leaves for flavouring.

Fennel is also well known for its medicinal value. It is most commonly associated with providing relief from various digestive disorders such as heartburn, bloating, colic in babies, respiratory tract infections, bedwetting, backache, and visual issues. Additionally, it is believed to promote milk secretion, ease birth, and promote menstruation. Fennel oil is used in beverages as a flavouring agent and in the manufacture of soaps and cosmetics for its fragrant component.

Fennel has a very rich history going back to ancient times. The Greeks called the herb *marathon* meaning 'grow thin' due to their belief in its ability to suppress appetite. The site of the well-known battle between Persians and Athenians in 490 BC is known by the name of Marathon, meaning the 'place of fennel'. Athenians even adapted the interwoven fennel stalks as their victory symbol. Prometheus, the Greek mythological figure who delivered fire to humanity, brought it hidden in a stalk of fennel.

In 812 AD (CE), Charlemagne declared that it should be grown in every garden as it had healing properties, and so he had it planted in the imperial gardens. The Roman philosopher, Pliny, is recorded to have said that fennel has the power to "take away the film that overcasts and dims our eyes"

During the 1200s, the fennel seed was used in England to suppress appetite and help people who were fasting to get through the long days. Later on it was commonly used during services to prevent stomach rumblings. In the 1700s the herb was used in a medical elixir, or tonic, known as absinthe, and not long after it was marketed as a spirit. It became popular with the Bohemians after WWI in the United States and Europe.

In the modern times, fennel seeds are easily available around the world in grocery stores, and the bulb in particular is well-liked in Europe.

Nutritional Value

Fennel is highly valued for its nutritional properties. It is low in sodium, saturated fat and cholesterol, and high in Vitamins C, Folate, Manganese, Calcium, Niacin, Potassium, Magnesium, Iron, Phosphorus, Copper and dietary fibre. It's phytonutrients with antioxidants have positive effects on health.

It's matchless amalgamation of unique phytonutrients like the flavonoids *rutin, querctin* and the *kaempferol glycosides,* are the ones responsible for their strong free radical eliminating activity. The uncontrolled free radicals are known to damage cells and lead to problems like osteoarthritis and rheumatoid arthritis.

The star phytonutrient found in fennel is anethole. This is the main component of fennel's oil. It is responsible for reducing swelling and putting off cancer. It is believed that anethole is useful for inhibiting the intercellular system of signals known as *tumour necrosis factor.* By closing down this system, activation of a gene changing and inflammation activating molecule is turned off and consequently these problems do not arise.

The bulb part of the fennel plant is a great source of vitamin C. This is the body's chief water-soluble antioxidant which can deactivate free radicals in every aqueous setting in the human body. The vitamin C found in fennel is antimicrobial which is required for the immune system's correct functioning.

The folate, a B vitamin found in fennel bulb, is responsible for converting the hazardous *homocysteine molecules* to harmless particles. At enhanced levels, homocysteine can damage blood vessels directly and is a substantial risk factor in heart attack and stroke. The bulb is also a source of fibre which is responsible for eliminating potentially cancer causing toxins from the colon. Hence, fennel can play a positive role in averting colon cancer.

Clinical Trials

Although it's a seemingly harmless condition, colic can be emotionally exhausting and physically tiring for parents. Thus far, dicyclomine hydrochloride is the only treatment that has worked effectively on a consistent basis. However, approximately 5% of the infants using it develop grave side effects, and at times even death. Clinical trials to determine the effect of fennel on colic babies were carried out in large multi-specialty clinics with 125 babies aged 2 to 12 weeks. The use of fennel oil provided relief to 65% of new-borns in the trial group[1].

In a placebo-controlled trial, the effect of fennel tea on chronic constipation was conducted on twenty randomly selected patients. There was noticeable improvement in the number of bowel movements and transit time through the colon. Effects were observed in the second day of treatment[2.] Because of the high levels of some constituents with known abilities to deter muscle cramps and muscle spasms, fennel seeds are chewed after meals in some cultures to prevent indigestion or gas.

Uses of fennel

Fennel seeds make a great flavouring agent in breads, cakes or cookies. The fresh leaves taste milder than the seeds and thus go well in salads, and soups. Alternatively, they can be chopped and added to fish or meat dishes. The stem and bulb part of the plant are good to sauté or roast, and used as side dishes. The bulbs also make a good addition for juicing recipes. Fennel's strong anise-

100

like flavour, make it a great choice for combining with celery, apples, or carrots in juicing recipes.

The use of fennel seeds does not require any special preparation. However, to extract the full aroma and accentuate the flavour, the seeds are best when toasted in a dry frying pan for a few minutes. Then they can then be crushed or ground before adding to the desired recipe. While toasting does slightly change the flavour, making it a bit spicier, it does not in any way alter the nutritional properties.

Fennel Tea - Preparation Method

- 1½ teaspoon of fresh crushed fennel seeds
- 1 cup of boiling water

Place the crushed seeds in a saucepan and then pour the boiling water over them. Allow the blend to seep for 7-10 minutes, being careful not it to boil a second time. Drink one cup of the tea three times a day after meals, to treat or prevent digestive issues such as bloating, gas, and heartburn. Drink the tea for four to six weeks to attain the desired effect.

Apple-Fennel Enchantment Juicing Recipe

- I medium sized Apple
- I bulb of fennel
- ¼ slice of ginger
- 2 carrots

In Mediterranean cooking, fennel is frequently enjoyed in the form of a marinated salad. A simple preparation that is sure to perk up any meal.

Cured Tangy Fennel Salad

- 1 cup of thinly sliced fresh fennel bulb
- Two teaspoons of olive oil
- ¼ teaspoon of lemon juice

- Salt & pepper to taste

Allow the mixture to marinate for several hours and serve at room temperature. Use a mandolin to get the slices as thin as possible.

Resources

1 http://www.ncbi.nlm.nih.gov/pubmed/12868253
2 Picon PD, Picon RV, Costa AF, et al. Randomized clinical trial of a phytotherapic compound containing Pimpinella anisum , Foeniculum vulgare , Sambucus nigra , and Cassia augustifolia for chronic constipation. BMC Complement Altern Med. 2010;10:17.

Figs

Introduction to Figs

Figs are a small, sweet and somewhat pear shaped fruit that grows on most of the over 1,000 Ficus tree species. Figs come in a range of varieties, sizes and colours. The raw fruit is consumed fresh from the tree and is considered to be very healthy however it may be dried or cooked as well.

Technically the fig is not a fruit but something classified as an in-frutescence. A genuine fruit is composed from a single plant ovum derived from a single blossom. An in-frutescence develops with multiple flower buds fusing together with the plant's sexual organs. Figs like pineapples are made from multiple ovaries and clusters of flowers joined together. In the majority of cases, the flowers blossom inside the fig giving rise to numerous seed pods that can be seen when the fruit is cut. Regardless of the technicalities, figs and pineapples are just called fruits.

Ficus carica is the common fig tree and one of the oldest cultivated plants known to man. So old in fact that it is even named in the Bible. The plant is not that big as far as trees go, reaching to a height of up to ten metres (33 ft.). It is ramified from the base with the crown possessing comparatively few branches. The buds of the plant are hairy with white, sticky latex like fluid. The leaves are roughly the size of a spread out hand with toothed edges, and 3 to 5 crested lobes. The bottom sides of the leaves have small hairs. Numerous small flowers develop on the plant.

History of Figs

According to a 2006 issue of Science magazine, University of Bar-Ilan researchers in Israel report parthenocarpic fig evidence at six Mediterranean region sites dating 11,700 and 10,500 years ago. This Pre-Potter Neolithic domestication evidence has been found at the sites of Jericho, Netiv Hagdud, Gilgal, Jordan Valley, Eurphrates Valley. Additionally fig remnants have been discovered at Neolithic excavation sites dating back to 5,000 B.C.E. Pliny knew of 29 varieties of figs.

Figs hold a prominent place in Greek mythology; they were presented as a gift to Dionysus by Demeter in return for the blessings of the Greek Gods. Greek athletes were documented by Plato as having been fed diets of figs to enhance running speeds and strength. Figs are 50% sugar, so it is akin to being fed a candy bar.

Figs also hold significance in all major religions of the world. The common fig is one of the two sacred plants mentioned in Islam. There is even a Sura in the Quran (the Holy Book of Mulsims) entitled "The Fig". Figs are also important in Buddhism, Hinduism and Jainism. According to tradition, the Bhudda is said to have found "bodhi" (enlightenment) meditating under the Sacred Fig tree (Ficus religiosa). The same species is the "world tree" of Hinduism. The common Fig is mentioned in the Bible in Genesis 3:7 when Adam and Eve used fig leaves to cover their nakedness and again in Mark 11:12-14 when Jesus cured a fig tree for not bearing fruit. The fig is one of the fruits promised in the Promised Land according to the Tora (Deut. 8).

Figs first appeared in England between 1525 and 1548. While it is not known exactly when they first entered China, it is known that they were established in Chinese gardens by 1550. The European fig plants were also taken to Japan, South Africa, India, China, and Australia.

Mexico was the first place where figs were planted in the New World and introduced to California in 1769 when the San Diego Mission was established. However, it was not until the 1900, when the wasp was instituted as the pollinating agent that commercial fig production became possible. Only the common fig is cultivated in India and the northern areas of South America and Florida, whereas other types better suited to cooler climates are cultivated in Chile and Argentina. Currently Turkey, Portugal, Greece, Spain and California are the largest fig producers.

Health Benefits of Figs

Figs contain a number of micronutrients that provide health benefits. Traditionally figs have been used to lower cholesterol, treat diabetes, constipation and a host of other disorders. Figs contain a high quantity of fibre which acts like a laxative in the body. Fibre adds mass and bulk which enhances regular bowel function and averts constipation. The elevated levels of fibre help to reduce weight and are frequently added to diets of obese people on a weight loss program. However, the high calorie count of the fruit can be counterproductive if too many are consumed; only a few figs are sufficient to get the job done. Figs also contain pectin, a soluble fibre that absorbs excessive lumps of cholesterol as it moves through the digestive system and removes them from the body, thus helping to lower cholesterol. The high levels of fibre in the diet are beneficial in averting abdominal, and colon cancers.

Figs are a source of phenol, Omega-3 and Omega-6 fatty acids, which play an active role in reducing the risk of coronary heart ailments. Additionally fig leaves have a direct effect on the triglyceride levels in the body. Fig leaves produce an inhibitory effect on triglycerides resulting in a drop in their numbers. Triglycerides are a major factor in a number of heart ailments. Fig leaves also cut down on the quantity of insulin required by insulin dependent diabetic patients. Fig leaf tea is typically employed to provide relief from respiratory conditions like bronchitis and asthma.

Additionally figs are a good source of potassium. This element helps in regulating the sugar absorbed by the body following a meal. Elevated amounts of potassium in the body reduce the blood sugar peaks and troughs experienced by diabetic patients and help them lead better lives. The high consumption of sodium through processed foods and low intake of potassium rich fruits and vegetables frequently leads to high blood pressure. The potassium rich and sodium deficient figs are perfect for averting effects of hypertension.

The abundant amount of calcium in figs is vital for good bone health and cutting down on the risks of osteoporosis. Furthermore the phosphorus in the fruit endorses bone formation and initiates regeneration if bones are damaged. The typically high sodium diets in today's society can lead to increased urinary calcium loss. The elevated amounts of potassium in figs regulate waste removal from the body. It averts the loss of calcium while enhancing the removal of toxic materials like uric acid.

Nutritional Benefits of Figs

Figs contain nominal amounts of saturated fats and sodium, and no cholesterol. They are high in dietary fibre. A 100 gram serving of fresh figs contains 80 calories, a little over one gram of protein, almost 2 grams of fibre and approximately 20 grams of carbohydrates. Same quantity of dried figs contains roughly three times the quantity of all these macronutrients.

In the micronutrient department, figs contain vitamins B1, B2 and B6, in addition to vitamins C, A, E and K. It also contains beta-carotene, choline and folate. Minerals found in figs include calcium, copper, iron, magnesium, manganese, phosphorous, selenium, potassium and zinc.

Uses of Figs

Almost all parts of the fig pant are usable. In addition to being consumed in teas, fig tree leaves are used to make a perfume with musk or wood aroma. The milky, white latex released by the tree can be used as a meat tenderizer or in cheese making by drying and powdering it.

Figs can be consumed out of hand. The more refined consumer however cuts the fig in halves peeling and discarding the skin and stem and consuming the flesh. In commercial preparations figs are peeled by dipping in boiling lye water for one minute or in boiling sodium bicarbonate solution. In more humid, warm climate, figs are consumed whole without peeling. Whole or sliced figs can be frozen for up to one year.

Figs can be stewed or cooked in a variety of ways in puddings, pies, cakes, breads and other bakery items. Additionally they may be used to make jam, marmalade or turned into a paste. The paste is used as filling in various bakery products. In Europe, California, northern Africa and west Asia commercial drying and canning of figs are significant industries. Dried, roasted, and ground figs are used as coffee substitute. The fruit can also be candied or dried for snacking purposes. In the Mediterranean countries the inferior quality figs are used to make alcohol. Alcoholic extracts are used as flavouring for tobacco and liqueurs.

Clinical Trials

One study involving 51,823 postmenopausal women showed a reduction in breast cancer risk for those eating the maximum amounts of fruit fibre as compared to those not eating it[1]. Additionally it has been found that figs contain phenolic compounds that play a positive role in human health in a number of ways. They do this by acting as antioxidants in a variety of ways such as free radical scavengers, hydrogen donators, reducing agents and more[2].

Extracts of *Ficus carica* showed elevated antibacterial activity against oral bacteria[3]. Fig latex agent has shown inhibitory effect against propagation of different types of cancer cells[4].

Resources

[1] http://www.ncbi.nlm.nih.gov/pubmed?Db=pubmed&Cmd=ShowDetailView&TermToSearch=17764112&ordinalpos=1&itool=EntrezSystem2.PEntrez.Pubmed.Pubmed_ResultsPanel.Pubmed_RVDocSum

[2] O. Çalişkan and A. Aytekin Polat, "Phytochemical and antioxidant properties of selected fig (Ficus carica L.) accessions from the eastern Mediterranean region of Turkey," Scientia Horticulturae, vol. 128, no. 4, pp. 473-478, 2011

[3] M.-R. Jeong, H.-Y. Kim, and J.-D. Cha, "Antimicrobial activity of methanol extract from Ficus carica leaves against oral bacteria," Journal of Bacteriology and Virology, vol. 39, no. 2, pp. 97-102, 2009

[4] S. D. Yancheva, S. Golubowicz, Z. Yablowicz, A. Perl, and M. A. Flaishman, "Efficient agrobacterium-mediated transformation and recovery of transgenic fig (Ficus carica L.) plants," Plant Science, vol. 168, no. 6, pp. 1433-1441, 2005

Garlic

According to folk medicine, garlic has the potential to cure everything from the common cold to the plague. While many of the old sayings are doubtful, prevailing scientific theories and research support numerous others. The main compounds that lend garlic its medicinal value are allicin and diallyl sulphides. The sulfur found in the garlic gives it the distinctive taste and medicinal value. Generally speaking, it has been found that the stronger the taste the greater the sulfur content, and consequently the greater the medicinal worth.

Garlic is perennial plant that was originally found in central Asia, but now cultivated throughout the world. It is a bulb-based vegetable belonging to the Allium class of plants, whose other members include leeks, onions, scallions and chives. The garlic plant can grow as tall as two feet or more, but it is the bulb part that is used in cooking and for medicinal purposes. The plant produces pink-purple flowers which bloom in the Northern Hemisphere from July to September. The bulb's outer layers contain a thin sheathing and the inner sheath holds the cloves. Each bulb consists of 4 to 20 segments, in a fully developed bulb.

The distinguishing flavour of garlic is due to the sulfuric content of the spice. This flavour is formed when the bioactive compound allicin is cut up or damaged. Garlic is a rich source of antioxidants, which help to remove free radicals from the body. Free radicals accumulate in the body with age and are a contributing factor to illnesses such as cancer, Alzheimer's and heart disease.

History

Garlic has held significance for almost every major society in the world. Its use has been noted in Egyptian and Chinese medicine for more than five thousand years. In fact, ancient Egyptians considered the herb so sacred that they even placed it in Pharaohs' tombs. The general concept is that garlic has the capacity to provide endurance and strength while offering protection from evil spirits. Greek and Roman athletes used garlic prior to taking part in a sports event, while soldiers took it before going off to battle. In fact it was even given to slaves building the Pyramids to help increase their stamina and strength.

In 1858, Louis Pasteur confirmed garlic's antiseptic characteristics and 'the father of medicine,' the Hippocrates, integrated garlic in treating cancerous tumours.

Garlic was valued for its antimicrobial results, long before the discovery of microbes. During the Middle Ages, French priests used garlic as protection against the bubonic plague, which we now know to be a bacterial infection. During World War I, garlic was applied directly to wounds by the European soldiers as a way to prevent infection. Today, garlic is recognized as an effective and safe preventive medicine in Europe. It is accepted by medical authorities as well as concerned government officials.

Nutritional Value

The bioactive components that make garlic valuable for health include arginine, oligosaccharides, selenium and flavonoids. It has especially low concentrations of saturated fats, sodium, natural sugars, and cholesterol. It has almost no calories (roughly four in each clove), and is loaded with vitamins A, B1, B2, B6, B12, C, D and E. The water soluble vitamin C and the fat soluble vitamin E are the two antioxidants responsible for the removal of free radicals from the body. Additional micronutrients that provide garlic with its healing usefulness, besides proteins and enzymes, include manganese, calcium, phosphorus, potassium, copper, and iron.

Health Benefits

Historically, garlic has been used to kill a wide range of microbes like viruses, fungi, parasites, and bacteria. Garlic is a good remedy against athlete's foot, viral diarrhoea, thrush (mouth infection caused by a fungus), and Helicobacter pylori, which is the bacteria responsible for causing ulcers. Other traditional applications of garlic include colds, flu, earaches, yeast infections, and elevated blood pressure.

Current research is focusing on four basic areas where garlic can be of benefit; heart disease, cancer, antioxidant properties, and infectious diseases. Studies involving cardiovascular issues and garlic have been conducted for more than three decades. Garlic lowers the LDL cholesterol levels by stopping the liver from producing excessive amounts of LDL. It does so without affecting the 'good' HDL cholesterol. It also plays the role of a blood thinner by decreasing the stickiness of platelets, thus preventing them from forming clots. This is vital for averting atherosclerosis, heart attacks, and stroke. Garlic slightly lowers blood pressure by dilating (widening) blood vessels. A critical review published in The Journal of Nutrition published in 2006 states that it has been established by scientists that cardiovascular disease benefits from garlic consumption.[1]

[2]Garlic is roughly 1% as powerful an antibiotic as penicillin, yet it is more successful against gram negative bacteria and without any of the side effects. Additionally, garlic seems to have immune stimulating, antioxidant, and liver protecting properties, but these properties have not as yet been that well investigated. Garlic has also shown promise when it comes to reducing pain related to rheumatoid arthritis, and has shown a reduction in the size of select cancerous tumours, but again further studies are required.

How to Use Garlic

There is plenty of evidence to indicate that garlic is beneficial as a preventive medicine. Including a minimum of half a clove to your food portion can yield positive results. If it is being cooked then 2-3 cloves should be used. For the majority of medicinal ailments, garlic is most beneficial when eaten raw. If eating it fresh is not acceptable, then add it to food towards the end of the cooking process, just before removing the heat, as this will help to retain the garlic's maximum amount of nutrients and flavour.

To eliminate the obvious odours associated with garlic it is possible to make tincture. Just peel one quarter pound of garlic cloves and allow seeping in half a quart of brandy. Seal and store for two weeks, not forgetting to shake thoroughly on a daily basis. Strain and take about thirty drops of the mixture daily.

When garlic is cooked, dried, or in the oil form, it loses a large portion of its potency. Peeled, chopped garlic, sold in stores has also lost a lot of its potency. Medicinal preparations should have at least 6,000 mcg of allicin to have the desired effect. While the supplements do not actually contain the allicin (as it is highly unstable and degenerates quickly), good supplements actually contain allin (allicin's precursor), which releases allicin upon digestion.

To use garlic as a cough syrup, and for relief from respiratory disorders, peel and slice one pound of garlic and submerge it in one quart of boiling water. Let the mixture stand for twelve hours. Add sugar or honey for a better taste until it reaches the consistency of syrup. Garlic tea, made by steeping a few cloves in a cup of water and left to stand overnight, is a great for sore throat.

Ointments for external wounds can also be prepared using garlic. Simply mash the clove into a fine paste and apply directly to the affected area. For ear aches, chop up a clove and lightly heat in a tablespoon of virgin olive oil. Allow the mixture to cool and strain. Add two to three drops of the solution in the affected ear three to four times a day.

Besides causing bad breath, no major side effects of garlic are known. Some minor reactions like nausea, flatulence, and bloating have been reported, and consuming a dose of 25ml of fresh garlic can produce a burning sensation in the mouth, stomach and esophagus. A few people are allergic to the herb. Finally, taking garlic simultaneously with certain types of medicine, such as those used to treat HIV/AIDS, carries potential risks to health. Also, consuming garlic in large doses carries the danger of postoperative bleeding. Hence, before embarking on a garlic regiment it is important to talk to your doctor and discuss all potential issues that may arise in your case.

Clinical Trials

Many studies involving medicinal properties of garlic are being carried out around the world. A number of population studies linking increased garlic consumption and a decrease in the possibility of developing cancers like colon, stomach, pancreas, breast, and oesophagus, have been carried out. An analysis of the results from seven such studies indicates the higher the quantity of raw and cooked garlic eaten, the lower the risk of colorectal cancer[3].

A number of studies carried out in China concentrated on the use of garlic and the risk of cancer. In one of these studies, it was found that oesophageal and stomach cancers had a lower risk of developing the cancer with greater consumption of garlic.[4] In another study, taking more than ten grams of allium vegetables like garlic reduced the risk of prostate cancer by roughly 50%.[5]

A randomised, placebo controlled study involving 146 subjects, tried to test whether garlic could actually prevent the common cold. Participants taking garlic every day for three months experienced fewer colds than those in the placebo group[6].

Resources

[1] Pubmed.gov, "Garlic and cardiovascular disease: a critical review." Rahman K. and Lowe GM. *Journal of Nutrition*. 2006 March; 136(3 Suppl): 736S- 740S.

[2] http://www.wright.edu/admin/fredwhite/pharmacy/popular_nremedies.html

[3] Fleischauer AT, Arab L. Garlic and cancer: A critical review of the epidemiologic literature. *Journal of Nutrition* 2001; 131(3s):1032S-1040S.

[4] Gao CM, Takezaki T, Ding JH, Li MS, Tajima K. Protective effect of allium vegetables against both esophageal and stomach cancer: A simultaneous case-referent study of a high-epidemic area in Jiangsu Province, China. *Japanese Journal of Cancer Research* 1999; 90(6):614-621.

[5] Hsing AW, Chokkalingam AP, Gao YT, et al. Allium vegetables and risk of prostate cancer: A population-based study. *Journal of the National Cancer Institute* 2002; 94(21):1648–1651.

[6] http://www.ncbi.nlm.nih.gov/pubmedhealth/PMH0013804/

Ginger

For many people the word 'ginger' brings to mind redheads with above average sexual drives, and exceptional fighting abilities. There is, however, another type of 'ginger' that people have been familiar with for a millennia. The herb is mentioned in the Koran, the Muslim holy book, indicating that the Arabs knew of the spice as early as 650 A.D. It is also spoken of in the writings of Confucius. Western Europeans have known about the spice since the 9th century.

A native of south eastern Asia, the rhizome's culinary properties were realized in the thirteenth century and its use became widespread all over Europe. It was a commonly traded plant during the renaissance and medieval times, and even though it was expensive, it was still in high demand. In the nineteenth century, barkeeper's kept containers of ground ginger handy for customers to sprinkle into their beer, which led to the origin of ginger ale.

General Information

The botanical name of ginger, *Zingiber Officinale,* is believed to have originated from its Sanskri name *Singabera*, meaning 'horn shaped'; an indication of its physical attributes. While repeatedly called 'ginger root', it is really a rhizome, a customized underground plant stem. Depending on the variety sewn, the flesh of ginger can be yellow, red, or white coloured. The skin is light brown in colour and can either be paper thin or fairly thick, depending on whether the plant is harvested when fully mature or still young.

Ginger is available in a variety of forms, but is best when used in its raw state. Dried ginger is available in two forms, as *black,* which still has the skin, and *white,* with the skin removed. Powdered ginger is made by grinding the dried root. The dried forms are not as aromatic and spicy as the fresh variety, nor are they as biting. Pickled ginger is cut up and preserved in a solution of spiced vinegar. Crystallized ginger is prepared by cooking the rhizome in sugary syrup, and then air drying before rolling it in sugar.

In the middle ages, it was recommended for nausea, hangovers, travel sickness and flatulence.[1] Ginger is officially a part of the pharmacopeias of China,

113

Austria, Egypt, India, Great Britain, Japan, Switzerland, and the Netherlands. It is used as a dietary supplement in the United States and has approval as a non-prescription drug in Germany.[2, 3]

Preparation & Serving Suggestions

Fresh ginger is prepared by removing the skin as one would remove the skin of an apple. The flesh can then be minced, sliced, or julienned. When the ginger is added during the cooking process, it affects the flavour of the dish. Added at the start it gives the dish a more subtle taste, but add it at the end and it delivers a stronger, more pungent taste.

Ginger is used around the globe in a variety of ways. In parts of the Middle East, the powdered form is used to spice up coffee, and in Egypt ginger is actually served in coffee shops. The traditional drink in Greece, called tsitsibira, is actually a type of ginger beer. In the Caribbean it is used in drink and food recipes. Ginger tea, made with fresh ginger, is a common beverage in Jamaica, while ginger beer is routinely made fresh in Jamaican homes. Western cuisine mostly employs ginger in sweet foods like gingerbread, biscuits, cakes, and ginger ale. In Japan and other places, pickled ginger is eaten between courses to clear the palate.

Here are a few unique ways to enjoy fresh ginger:

- Add a teaspoon full of fresh, grated ginger to a jug of lemonade and cool off. You can just chew on the small bits if you can tolerate the heat!
- Sprinkle half a teaspoon on top of rice for an exotic flavour and aroma.
- Perk up sautéed veggies by topping them off with fresh minced ginger.
- Add half a teaspoon of grated ginger to olive oil and garlic and dress up a salad for the perfect lunch treat.
- Grated ginger goes really well with the stuffing for baked apples.
- Fresh young ginger can be sliced and sprinkled into a salad. The more the quantity of the ginger in the salad the more spicy it becomes.

Ginger is packed with health promoting substances, and it is not necessary to use it in large quantities in order to get the full benefits. For example, ginger tea made with a couple of half inch slices, allowed to steep in a cup of hot water, is all that is required to settle an upset stomach. Arthritis patients have found relief consuming only a quarter inch slice of fresh ginger cooked in food. The majority of clinical trials use just 250 mg doses of ginger, three or four times a day.

Historical Health Benefits of Ginger

Ginger has been used for a long time in traditional Chinese medicine and Ayurvedic medicine in India. It is attributed with aphrodisiac properties according to the Karma Sutra, while employed in the Melanesian Islands to gain affection of the opposite sex. It is also a known diaphoretic, meaning it causes sweating. According to historical records, Henry VIII commanded that the spice should be used as plague medicine due to its diaphoretic properties. However, it is best known as a digestive aid. By the increased production of saliva and digestive fluids, it alleviates indigestion, diarrhoea, cramps, and pains caused by gas.

The rhizome is also well known for its anti-inflammatory characteristics. It aids by easing pain and reducing inflammation linked to arthritis, muscle spasms, and rheumatism. Its healing powers stimulate blood circulation, cleanse kidneys, remove toxins, and nourish the skin. Other curative uses include the treatment of respiratory conditions like asthma, and bronchitis, cut down on motion and morning sickness, treating nausea, and helping to break fevers by increasing perspiration.

Active ingredients responsible for its curative properties include gingerols, oleoresins, bisabolenel, zingibain, starch, essential oils like zingiberene, zingiberole, camphene, cineol, and borneol. The best thing about ginger is that there are hardly any side effects linked to it when taken in limited doses. Most frequently reported effects include bloating, heartburn, gas, and nausea, although these are usually linked with powdered ginger and not fresh.

Clinical Research

Recently ginger has attracted the attention of a lot of scientists. Clinical research is being carried out on the large variety of probable health benefits of the spice. A clinical research article published on January 4th, 2006, at the University of Michigan Comprehensive Cancer Center website, has shown that ginger has a lot of medicinal promise. Family medicine research investigator, Suzanna Zick, N.D., MPH, at the University of Michigan Health System, claims that use of ginger for ailments of the digestive tract and some types of arthritis has been promising[1].

Initial studies carried out at the Maryland Medical Center imply that ginger may also be beneficial in helping to lower cholesterol and act as a blood thinning agent[2]. In the controlled environment of a lab, studies indicate that the constituents of ginger possibly have anti-cancer properties. The American Cancer Society recognizes these medicinal properties of ginger, and recommends that it can be used as a medicine with caution. This is because it can extend bleeding when taken in combination with the typical blood thinning or clot preventing medicines. Even pregnant women with placental or other types of bleeding are asked by health care professionals to avoid using ginger during pregnancies.

Ginger has also been valued for its anti-inflammatory properties for centuries. It is, however, only over the past two and half decades that scientific proof has supplemented the belief that it contains anti-inflammatory constituents.[4] It is due to these anti-inflammatory components called gingerols, that people with osteoarthritis experience less pain and have greater mobility with regular use of ginger. Studies published in *Life Sciences* issue of November 2003 supports this, while a second study published in Journal of Alternative & Complementary Medicine in February 2005, show the mechanisms responsible for ginger's anti-inflammatory usefulness.

Ginger's sweat promoting properties are beneficial for treating colds and flu. Besides detoxifying, sweat contains germ-fighting agents that help to combat infections, according to German researchers. Dermicidin is the protein produced in the body's sweat glands, and transported to the skin with sweat, where it fights harmful bacteria like E. coli and staphylococcus aureus (responsible for skin infections), and fungi like Candida albicans.

Nutritional Value of Ginger

Ginger is free of cholesterol and low in calories. It is also an excellent source of vitamins and other micronutrients. It contains foliates, niacin, pantothenic acid (vitamin B5), Pyridoxine (vitamin B6), vitamins A, C, E, and K. Additionally it is rich in electrolytes like sodium and potassium and minerals like calcium, copper, iron, magnesium, manganese, phosphorus and Zinc. Finally, it is a source of dietary fibre, carbohydrates and protein.

Resources

1. http://www.cancer.med.umich.edu/news/gingerhm06.shtml

2. http://umm.edu/health/medical/altmed/herb/ginger#ixzz2iiGr3bKK

3. Langner E, Greifenberg S , Gruenwald J . Ginger: history and use. Adv Ther. 1998; 15(1):25-44.

4. Blumenthal M, Busse W, eds. German Commission E Monographs: Therapeutic Monographs on Medicinal Plants for Human Use. Austin, TX: American Botanical Council; 1997.

5. Newall C, et al. Herbal Medicines: A Guide for Healthcare Professionals. London: Pharmaceutical Press; 1996.

6. Ginger--an herbal medicinal product with broad anti-inflammatory actions.Grzanna R, Lindmark L, Frondoza CG.RMG Biosciences, Inc. *J Med Food*. 2005 Summer; 8(2):125-32.

Grapefruit

Citrus paradise, or better known as the grapefruit, grows on a subtropical citrus tree belonging to the Rutaceae family. It is available today in a number of varieties distinguished by the colour of the fruit's pulp, which can range from red, white, to hues of pink. The colouration is a result of pigmentation and the stage of ripeness. The fruit taste ranges from sharp acidic, to lightly bitter, and sweet or sour. The fruit can also be mildly fragrant, with the skin being totally yellow, or a hue of pink with yellow. Mercaptan, a terpene with sulfur, is among the materials responsible for the taste and fragrance of grapefruit.

Other than for consumption as a fruit, grapefruits are used in a number of commercial productions. Grapefruit juice is used for medicinal purposes against a large range of ailments. The seed extract is also orally consumed for its medicinal properties. Additionally, the extract is used as a facial cleanser, remedy against mild skin irritations, and a dental rinse for healthy gums. Its oil is applied to the scalp to enhance hair growth, and to the skin for treating acne, oily skin, and muscle fatigue. In manufacturing, grapefruit seed extracts and oil provide a delicate scent in soaps, household cleaners, and cosmetics. In agriculture, the seed extracts are employed to destroy bacteria, fungus and moulds, preserve food, kill parasites in animal feed, and disinfect water. The peel of the fruit is used in aromatherapy.

History of Grapefruits

Griffith Hughes was the first person to describe the grapefruit in 1750, calling it the "forbidden fruit" of Barbados. Later in 1789, Patrick Browne noted that it was growing all over Jamaica, and he too described it as the "forbidden fruit" and also "smaller shaddock". A number of botanists believe the fruit was the result of a natural breeding process between an orange and the pomelo (another citrus fruit that came to Barbados from Indonesia in the 17th century). In 1814, John Lunan described it as a variety of shaddock albeit significantly smaller. At around this time it was given the name of grapefruit, a reflection of the way in which the fruit hangs in clusters like grapes.

It was in 1823 that Count Odette Phillipe carried the fruit's seeds to Tampa, Florida. Upon the fruiting of these initially planted grapefruits, the first generations of these newly developed seeds were passed around the neighbourhood. Initially the plants were grown merely for ornamental purposes. In 1870, John A. MacDonald became so enticed by a single grapefruit tree with it clusters of fruit he saw growing on a private property, that he purchased the entire crop. He then planted its seeds, thus establishing the very first grapefruit nursery on his property. George W. Bowen planted the very first grove using the seedlings from this nursery in 1875, and started to develop the fruit on a commercial basis. Eventually the commercial production of the grapefruit spread to other countries like Israel, South Arica, and Brazil.

Health Benefits of the Grapefruit

The grapefruit is an outstanding source of a number of phytochemicals that contribute to a healthy diet. Over the years a large portion of the populace has endorsed the fruit for its ability to burn fat. It is a good weight-loss diet food due to having less than one hundred calories and high, hunger quenching fibre content. Researchers at the Scripps Clinic in California, USA claim that by consuming half a grapefruit prior to each meal may help a person lose up to one pound a week, even when there are no other changes made in diet. Ken Fujioka, MD, the author of the study, claims that a compound found in grapefruits helps to regulate insulin and anything that lowers insulin aids in lowering weight[1].

Grapefruit is thought to be valuable in the treatment of influenza and malaria. The 'naringin' found in the fruit, and responsible for its bitter taste, helps to neutralize acidity, and is also thought to be a flavonoid with powerful antioxidant properties. Antioxidants have antiviral, antibacterial, antifungal, anti-cancer, and anti-inflammatory properties, which enhance the immune system and protect against influenza. Additionally, it contains natural 'quinine', a substance with a history of treating malaria, along with arthritis, lupus and nocturnal cramps in legs.

Nootkatone is a highly valuable compound when it comes to extraction of aromatic substances, but more importantly it improves metabolism in the body resulting in greater levels of energy and endurance. Hence, grapefruits are good for fighting fatigue. Grapefruits also aid indigestion due to the high fibre and vegetative pulp content. The fruit improves the flow of digestive juices, thereby, easing bowel movement and regulating excretory system.

Grapefruits are good for diabetics. Consumption of grapefruit brings down the amount of starch in the body, thereby regulating sugar levels in the blood. A glass of grapefruit before bedtime aids insomnia. The chemical 'tryptophan' is associated with making one sleepy after consuming a big meal, and is also present in grapefruits. Grapefruit membranes are full of pectin, a soluble fibre that helps to lower cholesterol.

Nutritional Value

Grapefruits are jam packed with nutrients. They have over 60 phytonutrients, with many flavonoids. This class of antioxidants is believed to fight allergies, infections, heart disease, ulcers, and cancer. Exact nutritional value of grapefruits varies with the variety of the fruit (pink, red or white), with the pink and red varieties having greater amounts of vitamin A, full range of B vitamins (except B-12) and folic acid. A half grapefruit supplies more than 50% of the Recommended Dietary Allowance of vitamin C. Just one cup of fresh grapefruit provides 1 gram of protein, 3 grams of fibre, and between 17 to 22 grams of carbohydrates. Additionally, it contains calcium, potassium, phosphorous, iron, zinc, and magnesium.

Individuals on synthetic man-made drugs have to proceed with caution when it comes to regular use of grapefruits. It contains elevated levels of the flavonoid naringin which rejects such drugs. The flavonoid is a useful substance under normal conditions. It recognizes foreign composites that should not be present in the body and thus deals with them as toxins. It also treats the synthetic drugs as toxins and halts their metabolism, leaving them in the body and enhancing the risk of toxic poisoning. For people not using any medications, grapefruit is a very healthy fruit to use on a regular basis. However, for those on medication, it is best to consult a doctor before using grapefruit regularly.

How to Use a Grapefruit

It is best to first wash grapefruits under cool water to remove any dirt or pesticide deposits. Even in cases where the peel is not going to be consumed;

cutting unwashed fruit can transfer dangerous substances into the flesh. Grapefruits may be eaten like oranges, or they can be sliced horizontally into halves and the flesh scooped out with a spoon. Alternatively, they can be sliced vertically, and the skin peeled off with fingers or a knife.

Segments of the fruit may be added to green or fruit salads.

The juice of grapefruit is very refreshing on its own or when mixed with other juices.

It is used in jams, desserts, marmalades and jellies.

Its peel is candied and is a vital source of pectin used in preserving other fruits.

As a matter of course grapefruit is a breakfast fruit. It's traditionally cut in half with the individual sections loosened using a special grapefruit knife and the pulp is spooned out of the shell. It can be sweetened with either brown sugar or honey. For additional benefits, cinnamon or nutmeg may be sprinkled on top. It can also be used as an appetizer before dinner; again served by separating the fruit in two halves horizontally, sweeten lightly, broiled, and served hot with a maraschino cherry on top.

The peel oil is commonly used as flavouring in soft-drinks after removing half of the monoterpenes. Nootkatone is the major component of the outer peel. It is extracted and added to powdered grapefruit juice to enhance the flavour of the reconstituted juice. Naringin is extracted from the inner peel and used in bitter "tonic" beverages, ice creams, and chocolates. It is also converted to a sweetener that is roughly 1,500 times as sweet as normal sugar.

Clinical Trials

According to a new study, a glass of grapefruit juice allows patients to get the same advantage from anti-cancer medicines as they would if they consumed three times as much of the drug on its own. This will help reduce the cost medicines over long term use[2].

In another study, it was found that nanoparticles obtained from grapefruits can be used to deliver drugs to specifically targeted locations. This technique can prove to be an inexpensive mode of making customized treatments. Currently they are being tested in clinical trials for safety in colon cancer patients[3].

Resources

[1] http://www.medicalnewstoday.com/releases/5495.php

[2]http://www.uchospitals.edu/news/2012/20120807-sirolimus.html

[3]http://nih.gov/researchmatters/june2013/06032013grapefruit.htm

Grapes

Introduction to Grapes

Other than Antarctica, grapes are grown on every continent of the world. Grapes (*Vitis vinifera*) are actually classified as berries. They come in round or oval shapes and have juicy semi-transparent flesh inside. They grow in clusters ranging from six to three hundred fruits with most common varieties being green, red or purple/black in colour. They have a sour taste when not yet ripe due to the malic acid they contain, but as they ripen the content of the acid decreases and they become sweet tasting. They have to be hand-picked as machines tend to bruise them easily. Grapes serve three primary uses: for wine production, as dried fruit (raisins) and as fresh fruit.

The fruits develop on robustly climbing vines which can reach the height of fifteen to twenty five metres if left without pruning. The deciduous vine (leaves lost in winter) has flat green leaves that are lightly lobed and have saw like edges. The thin snake-like tendrils secure the vine by twisting around any available structure and support the plant as it climbs higher. Wild grape vines are able to even climb over trees and block sufficient sunlight from reaching the trees to kill them. The flowers produced develop in clusters and are small, green and have a fragrance. Clusters of grapes develop from the fertilized flowers.

History of Grapes

Wild grapes have been around almost as long as civilization itself. They are believed to have originate somewhere in East Europe, Middle East or North Africa. Some evidence suggests that grapes were grown as early as 6500 B.C in the Neolithic era. Around 4000 B.C.E. grape cultivation extended into Asia Minor and along the Nile Delta of Egypt.

The Hittites were responsible for spreading grapes westward as they journeyed to Crete, Thrace and Bosporus as long ago as 3000 B.C.E. The Phoenicians and Greeks promoted the growth of the fruit to Sicily, Carthage, Spain and France. The Romans took charge and spread it further throughout all of Europe.

Man learned of the art of fermentation and converting grapes into wine in the Stoneage. Egyptians were the first people to produce wine. However at that time it was not used for social drinking. It was mainly employed in religious ceremonies and temple rituals. The Greeks and Romans grew grapes for use as substitutes for sugar. They produced syrups like passum, and sapa, which were then used to flavour dishes. Syrups made from grapes are still common in Levant regions and Turkey.

Towards the end of the Roman Empire, wine production was mainly associated with monasteries. Later on its use went beyond the religious boundaries and it became a part of the social culture. With this the demand for grapes continuously grew from the 16th century to date. King Hammurabi of Babylon is believed to be the initiator of the very first liquor law when he set down the rules for trading wine in 1700 B.C.E.

Health Benefits of Grapes

Grapes are only tiny in size but they are big when it comes to delivering health benefits. While all varieties of grapes are good for health, the darker coloured ones tend to offer greater benefits. This is because grapes with darker skin, namely red and purple/black ones have a higher content of resveratrol. This polyphenol found in grape skin is a natural anti-pathogenic that is believed to block cell signals through what is known as the Writ pathway. This pathway is connected with more than 85% of sporadic colon cancers. Reveratrol has also be shown to be effective in treating skin and gastrointestinal cancers in addition to suppressing tumours of lung, breast, prostate and leukaemia.

Resveratrol also works to clean out brain damaging plaques and free radicals found in patients suffering from Alzheimer's disease. Grapes delay the onset of degenerative neural diseases. According to a study published in the British Journal of Nutrition, grapes can even improve brain function in people who already have minor cognitive impairment[1].

Grapes also contain the powerful bioflavonoid, quercetin which works with vitamin C to accelerate the immune system to combat infection, inflammation, and cancer in addition to providing relief from anguishing pain for arthritis and gout patients. Grapes added to a diet help to maintain alkalinity. When blood and urine are a little more alkaline, acidic wastes are removed from the body more easily leading to fewer attacks of painful rheumatoid arthritis and recurring gout symptoms. Uric acid crystals that form with reduced kidney function dissolve easily in alkaline urine and are eliminated from the body thus averting their deposit in joints of gout patients.

The University of Michigan Cardiovascular Centre made grape powder mixture using red, green and black grapes inclusive of seeds and skin. They added this powder to the diet fed to the rats. After eighteen weeks the rats given the grape enriched diet had less inflammation, lower blood pressure, better heart function and fewer signs of heart damage compared to the rats that had the same diet without grape powder enrichment.

Nutritional Value of Grapes

Grapes have an amazing composition of phytonutrients like poly-phenolic antioxidants, vitamins and minerals. They are low in saturated fat, sodium and cholesterol. They are a good source of Vitamin K and C. They also have small amounts of vitamin A and E, niacin, folates, pantothenic acid, pyridoxine, riboflavin, and thiamine. They contain small amounts of the electrolyte potassium and trace amount of sodium. In the mineral department they are a good source of copper, small amounts of calcium, iron, magnesium, manganese, and trace amount of zinc.

The large variety of phytonutrients in grapes make them a powerhouse for good health. While no single variety contains all of the mentioned micronutrients, grapes in general provide Flavanols like catechins, epicatechins, and procyanidins, Flavonols like quercetin , kaempferol , and myricetin. They also contain important Carotenoids like beta-carotene, lutein, zeaxanthin and Phenolic Acids such as caffeic acid, coumaric acid, and ferulic acid.

Uses of Grapes

Freshly purchased grapes can stay in the refrigerator for up to 5 to 7 days. Before eating them, make sure to wash them thoroughly to remove any possible pesticide remains. For best flavour, grapes should be served slightly chilled. But, grapes are not for just eating out of hand, you can make jams, jellies and preserves out of them, use them in baking, or fresh salads, juice them on their own or in combination with other fruits. For long term preservation grapes can be canned, or frozen.

Frozen grapes make a great summertime treat. Just remove the grapes from the vines and after washing, spread them on a cookie sheet to freeze. Frozen in this way they can be eaten as a snack or used in salads or added to yogurt like fresh grapes. They keep their shape remarkably well when defrosted. Juiced grapes, sweetened lightly with honey can make great popsicles.

Clinical Trials

A number of related conditions including high blood sugar, blood pressure, extra fat around waist, elevated cholesterol that lead to chronic diseases are known as metabolic syndrome. Researchers at the University of Michigan presented a paper at the Experimental Biology Conference showing grapes protect damage to organs linked with advancement of metabolic syndrome. They believe the polyphenols in grapes are responsible for this effect. The team claims consuming grapes of different coloured varieties can have major impact on metabolic syndrome[2].

Macular degeneration is a condition where the centre of the retina, called the macula, deteriorates and is one of the main causes of blindness in the aged. A study published in Free Radical Biology and Medicine claims that consumption of grapes during one's lifetime can aid in slowing or preventing this age-linked condition. It is thought that the action of antioxidants in grapes is the cause of this protective effect. Antioxidants form a protective shield to protect against repeated exposure to high intensity sun light and may avert blindness[3].

University of Illinois researchers reported the resveratrol found in grapes halts the growth of tumours at all stages, while France's Liver Research Study Group says that resveratrol stops liver cancer by blocking tumour cell invasion[4].

Complutense University of Madrid, Spain researchers extracted Grape Antioxidant Dietary Fibre (GADF) from seeds and skin of red grapes and added it to meals of 34 adults. After sixteen weeks, it was found that the group taking GADF showed a five percent decrease in blood pressure, and a fourteen percent decrease in cholesterol. High cholesterol patients who consumed GADF also registered a reduction of over fourteen percent in total cholesterol and over eleven percent decrease in LDL (bad) cholesterol[5].

Resources

[1]http://journals.cambridge.org/download.php?file=%2FBJN%2FBJN103_05%2FS0007114509992364a.pdf&code=dc6a46edeb9fe0ef6cb278dbfe6e39fd

[2]http://www.naturalnews.com/040344_grape_extract_metabolic_syndrome_grapes.html

[3]http://www.naturalnews.com/034949_grapes_blindness_AMD.html

[4]http://www.naturalnews.com/028801_grapes_gout.html

[5]http://www.naturalnews.com/025654_cholesterol_diet_disease.html

Green Beans

Introduction to Green Beans

French beans, green beans, string beans and snap beans, are actually different names of the same bean scientifically known as *Phaseolus vulgaris*. The beans are made up of a green pod with tiny seeds inside and range in size from four to six inches. The pod and the seeds inside are consumed as a single unit. The term "string bean" was born out of the customary preparation exercise of eradicating a string like fibre from the pod before cooking. However, the new varieties of the vegetable no longer have the strings and the only preparation needed is to snap off the ends.

There are two chief subdivisions of green beans known as bush and pole beans. Bush beans develop on short plants that reach the height of roughly two feet and do not require any support. They tend to attain maturity and produce fruit in a fairly short period of time, and then cease fruit production. Due to this, more than a single crop of bush beans can be cultivated in a season. Pole beans grow on plants that grow much taller and require support of poles, hence the name.

There are more than 130 varieties of green beans. Typically used varieties are usually selected for their flavour, succulence and pods and are frequently grown in home gardens. Pod colour can range from green to purple, red or streaked. Even the pod shapes show variation from thin strips like "fillet" to wider "romano" styles and a whole range in between.

History of Green Beans

The green bean originates in Central and South America and was domesticated in ancient times. Seeds of the cultivated varieties have been found in deposits in Peru. Columbus introduced the green bean to the Mediterranean upon return from his second voyage to the New World in 1493. By the seventeenth century, the green bean was cultivated widely in Italy, Greece and Turkey. The largest producers of green beans today are Argentina, Egypt, China, France, India, Indonesia, Italy, Iraq, Spain, Mexico, Netherlands and U.S.A.

A classic American comfort food, the green bean casserole is a staple dish at Thanksgiving dinners. The casserole was the brain child of Dorcas Reilly of Campbell Soup Company, who wanted to ensure that her cream of mushroom soup kept selling. She came up with the quick to make dish with ingredients that would be easily available in most American homes, and the dish was born. Requiring only a few ingredients and easily adjustable to varying tastes, the dish is very easy to make. The original green bean casserole recipe belonging to Dorcas Reilly now sits in the National Inventors Hall of Fame on a yellowing 8 X 11 recipe card along with Thomas Edison's light bulb.

Health Benefits of Green Beans

Green Beans are loaded with dietary fibre, nearly 9% in each 100 gram serving. The fibre behaves like a laxative, protecting the mucous membrane of the large intestine by minimizing the exposure to toxic substances and binding with cancerous chemicals in the colon. Additionally it aids in lowering bad cholesterol in the body. People afflicted with diabetes can also benefit from green beans as fibre helps to regulate blood sugar levels.

The high levels of vitamin A in green beans, along with flavonoid poly-phenolic antioxidants like zea-xanthin, lutein and ß-carotene together act as scavengers of oxygen-derived free radicals. This helps to protect against heart disease, cholesterol and cancer. The vitamin A also postpones premature ageing by reducing wrinkles, dark spots, and fine lines. The Zea-xanthin in green beans is absorbed by the retinal macula in the eyes and provides UV filtering functions as well as antioxidant activity. Hence green beans offer protection against the age related macular disease (ARMD) in the aged.

In case of injury, the vitamin K helps the body to heal faster by hastening the process of blood clotting. It also allows for more calcium to be absorbed by the body which promotes bone health and density. This reduces the chances of developing osteoporosis. Additionally it is beneficial to women with iron deficiencies. Vitamin C also aids in healing wounds and might have a role in cancer prevention. The antioxidant characteristics of vitamin C protect cellular DNA from damage. The manganese in green beans, besides lessening the symptoms of osteoporosis also helps other nutrients to be absorbed by the body. The significant amounts of silicon in green beans reinforce connective tissue and bone health.

It is a misconception that green beans do not provide sufficient amounts of pigments like carotenoids. Recent studies indicate that lutein, beta-carotene, violaxanthin, and neoxanthin which tomatoes and carrots are so well recognized for are also present in green beans. In fact their quantities are comparable[1].

Nutritional Value of Green Beans

Green beans can be consumed in a variety of ways but to get the maximum nutritional benefits, cook them only lightly. Over cooking green beans diminishes some of their nutritional value, especially vitamin C and minerals. While a one hundred gram serving of cooked green beans and raw beans have the same amount of protein, B vitamins, as well as vitamins A and E, cooking wastes approximately thirty percent of the iron, potassium and magnesium and twenty percent of vitamin C.

A one hundred gram serving of raw green beans provide only 31 calories, roughly 7 grams of carbohydrates, 3 grams dietary fibre and 2 grams protein. It contains less than a quarter gram of fat. In the vitamin department the one hundred gram serving delivers 15% vitamin C, 14% vitamin K, 11% vitamin B6, 9% vitamin B2, 8% folate, 7% vitamin B1, 5% vitamins B3 and B5 and 4% vitamin A.

Green beans also contain a good range of some important minerals. A one hundred gram serving delivers 10% of the daily recommended allowance of manganese (based on a 2000 calorie diet), 8% iron, 7% magnesium, 5% phosphorus, 4% each of potassium and calcium, 3% zinc and trace amounts of fluoride.

Uses of Green Beans

While over cooking does destroy some of the nutrients in green beans, steaming for five minutes does no harm. Cooked in this way, they retain their crispness along with most of their nutrients. If frozen initially and then steamed as described, green beans still retain most of their nutrients. Canned green beans lose roughly one third of their phenolic compounds in the canning process, along with some vital B vitamins.

Some quick ideas for using green beans include:

- Throw a handful into stir fries.
- Add to curries and soups.
- Sauté with mushrooms.
- Throw together some raw green beans with a clove of ground garlic, some olive oil, feta cheese and slivered almonds for a great tasting side dish.
- They go well in grilled-salads.

Snap Crackle Green Beans
Ingredients:

- ½ kg green beans
- 1/4 cup buttermilk
- 1/2 cup flour
- 1/4 cup cornmeal
- 1 tsp. baking powder
- 2 tsp. salt plus more for sprinkling
- 1/4 tsp. cayenne (optional)
- Oil for frying

Preparation

1. Wash and totally dry the green beans. Place them in a bowl and add the buttermilk to just coat them.
2. Combine flour, cornmeal, baking powder, salt, and cayenne in a large bowl. Drain the extra buttermilk, and add the green beans to the flour mixture, coat well.
3. Heat about 1/2 inch of oil well over medium heat in a wide, heavy pot.
4. Shake the extra flour mixture off the beans and add so there is a single layer in the frying pot. Fry until beans are tender and reach a golden to medium brown colour.

Clinical Trials

According to recent studies the nutritional value of green beans has be highlighted even more. When compared to other foods in the bean family, green beans were found to come out on top. It is now confirmed that in addition to antioxidants like flavonoids quercetin and kaemferol they also contain catechins, epicatechins, and procyanidins. Green beans also contain carotenoids like lutein, beta-carotene, violaxanthin, and neoxanthin[1].

In a study conducted over six years, researchers found diets rich in green and yellow vegetables slow the development of atherosclerosis, which means it might lead to lowering the risk of coronary heart disease. In the study, mice were divided into two groups, one being fed a diet without vegetables and the other group was given a blend of green vegetables including green beans for 16 weeks. It was found that aortic atherosclerosis was lowered by 38%[2].

Resources

[1]http://whfoods.org/genpage.php?tname=btnews&dbid=144

[2]http://www.ncbi.nlm.nih.gov/pubmed/16772454

Jicama

Introduction to Jicama

Jicama or *Pachyrihizus erosus,* an edible root bearing a resemblance to turnips, is a member of the Fabaceae family. A native of Mexico, its other names include yam bean, Mexican potato, or Mexican turnip. All parts of the plant that are above the ground, including flowers, seeds, pods, vine and leaves, contain the compound rotenone which makes them toxic. The root is the only part of the plant that is safe for human consumption. Two main varieties of the vegetable exist. The agua is shaped like a turnip and yields translucent juice. It is the preferred, more commonly available variety in markets. Leche has an elongated shape and produces milky juice.

Jicama vines can reach 20 to 30 feet in size when fully mature, and grow vigorously in tropical and semitropical climates. The leaves are rhomboid to egg shape with toothed edges and extend up to six inches in length. The violet to white flowers lead the way for seed pods which are five to six inches long. The tubers are brown skinned with crisp white flesh. The nutty tasting, mildly sweet, crunchy tuber offers numerous culinary uses.

The jicama root, if allowed, can grow to unbelievable sizes. In 2010 in the Philippines (where they are known as singkamas), the heaviest recorded jicama weighed in at 23 kg! In Central America the root is sold by street vendors for raw eating, seasoned with lime or lemon juice and chilli powder. Other than Central America, the root is popular in South Asia, Caribbean and a few Andean South American regions.

History of Jicama

Jicama has origins in Mexico, Central and South America. It has been grown by all the major civilizations of the region and has constituted an important part of the staple diet. In the seventeenth century it was introduced to the Philippines by the Spanish, and from there it found its way into Southeast Asia and China. Jicama was used as a staple food onboard trading ships due to the fact that it had a long storage life. Additionally it could be eaten raw and served as a good thirst quencher. It is most commonly used in Mexico, South China and the U.S now.

Health Benefits of Jicama

There are a great many health benefits associated with jicama consumption. Whether you cook it or eat it raw, it delivers a number of vital nutrients that are essential to good health. Jicama is also found as an ingredient in a number of products like scrubs, masks, moisturizers, lotions and facial soaps. The high content of water provides a moisturizing effect. The saponins in it behave as a natural sunscreen and avert skin damage to prevent wrinkles and improve skin texture. The phenolic compounds prevent the production of melanin, meaning pigmentation resulting from hormones, acne scars and sunlight is minimized. Being rich in vitamin C, jicama shows properties of an antihistamine and enhances the immune system. It behaves like an anti-inflammatory and is highly beneficial for individuals suffering from asthma. It is also used to treat common colds and flu.

It is considered to be a very good source of inulin, a pre-biotic that enhances the growth of good bacteria in the intestines. The dietary fibre in Jicama speeds up the movement of waste in the digestive tract, and aids in its expulsion from the body. The minimal pressure and pain with smooth elimination of waste from the body leads to relief from haemorrhoids. Drinking juice of jicama each morning can be beneficial to people suffering from the ailment. The fibre also aids in lowering cholesterol and maintains blood sugar levels. This is because it is not converted into glucose and moves out of the system at a steady pace. It gives the feeling of being full longer, thus helping to maintain a healthy weigh.

Homocysteine is an amino acid associated with higher risks of heart disease due to its ability to reduce the blood vessel lining. Present in large quantities in meats, it is also linked to renal disease. Jicama contains anti-homocysteine properties. According to some figures, regular use of this veggie reduces the quantity of this amino acid by 11%, which in turn reduces the risks of heart disease.

Nutritional Value Jicama

Jicama is considered to be a good food because it contains no saturated fat or cholesterol, very little sodium and only a few calories and yet it delivers plenty of good things like fibre, vitamins and minerals. It also provides some protein. One cup of uncooked jicama offers 40% of daily recommended amount of vitamin C. It also provides 5% of the daily potassium requirement, 4% manganese, iron and magnesium, 3% copper, 2% phosphorus, and 1% calcium, zinc and selenium.

Uses of Jicama

To prepare jicama, just wash them thoroughly under cool running water and wipe dry. Remove the thick fibrous skin with a vegetable peeler or a paring knife. The peel and all other plant parts contain rotenone, an organic poison, so discard those. The pure white flesh can now be cubed, grated, sliced or chopped.

One of the best ways to eat jicama is on its own and raw. Just dress the cut up veggie with a little chilli powder and sprinkle with lime juice and a pinch of salt. It can be consumed in a variety of more complex ways like soups and salads or as a baked, boiled, steamed, micro waved side dish to a main course. Jicamas can take the place of apples, pears or water chestnuts in recipes. Advocates of raw food employ the jicama in green drinks due to the high vitamin c and enzyme content.

Some Quick Serving Methods
- Make a Jicama Combo with cubed jicama, cucumber and orange segments. Season with salt, lemon juice and chilli powder.
- They make great additions to stir fries.
- Roast jicama by cutting them into cubes and mixing with chopped onion. Mix with a few teaspoons of olive oil, ½ teaspoon of ground garlic, and sprinkled with rosemary and parsley. Bake the mixture on a cookie sheet at 400 degrees until the pieces are tender.
- Make relish with jicama to use on burgers
- Jicama coleslaw also comes out great.

Jicama chips

- Peel and thinly slice jicama
- Individually place the slices on a paper towel to allow extra moisture to be removed.
- Heat peanut oil and fry the jicama slices until golden brown.
- Drain on a paper towel to remove excess oil.

The chips can be enjoyed as they are or they can be topped with Italian seasoning and parmesan cheese.

Clinical Trials

Phytoestrogen is a plant-derived natural alternative that shows potential in preventing bone loss. A non-steroid that is very nearly like estrogen and has estrogenic and antiestrogenic properties has shown promising results in protecting against bone loss due to estrogen deficiency[1].

Japanese researchers have found jicama fibre to be of benefit in the immune system[2]. The prebiotic inulin has tummy flattening properties and helps to elevate the friendly bacteria found in the digestive tract and might aid in eliminating wrinkles through the increased production of collagen.

Resources

[1] http://www.arjournals.org/index.php/ijpm/article/viewFile/132/124

[2] http://health.yahoo.net/experts/dayinhealth/seven-newest-superfoods

Jerusalem artichokes

Introduction to Jerusalem artichokes

Although it goes by the name of Jerusalem artichoke, it has absolutely no connection with Jerusalem nor does it have any relation to the true artichoke! It is actually more closely related to the sunflower. According to one school of thought, the word Jerusalem is derived from the Italian word 'girasole' meaning 'turning toward the sun' just like the sunflower does. Another thought is that 'Artichoke' is a distortion of the Arabic word 'al-khurshuf,' relating to its out of the ground foliation. Yet another thought claims it is a distortion of the 'Ter Neusen,' the part of Netherlands from where it was initially launched into Europe.

The vegetable also goes by the names of sun-root and sun-choke. The lumpy tuber has light brown skin, looks like ginger root and has a crunchy, nutty sweet taste similar to that of chestnuts. It develops underground like the potato, however, it is more difficult to harvest as the tubers become entangled with the roots sticking to them. In the wild varieties, sun chokes mature at the end of the root, while in the cultivated varieties they develop as clumps near the main rhizome. Similar to the sunflower, the sun-choke plant can grow from three to twelve feet in height. The plant's flowers are one and a half to three inches in diameter with large leaves. Sun-choke plants tend to behave like weeds by multiplying and taking over the area in which they are grown.

History of Jerusalem artichokes

Artichoke is a native of North America and grew in the wild along the east coast from Georgia to Nova Scotia. Samuel de Champlain, an explorer, first discovered the vegetable growing in the garden of an indigenous American Indian in Massachusetts in 1605. He thought they tasted like artichokes, and took them back to France. The natives called them sun roots and introduced them to the pilgrims when they landed on the continent. The perennial tuber was incorporated into the pilgrim's diet as a staple food. The Italians were introduced to the veggie prior to 1632, and got to know it as 'girasole.'

The rise to popularity of the vegetable was quick in the 1600, perhaps due to the name of artichoke associated with it. At this time the potato was not that well accepted. As the potato rose in fame, Jerusalem artichoke fell from grace. The public somehow got the idea that it was responsible for causing leprosy. Part of the reason for this thought was its awkward shape and blotchy brown skin that gave the appearance of the distorted fingers of people suffering from leprosy.

It wasn't until 1772 when Europe was hit with famine that Jerusalem artichoke was turned to for sustenance. It was easy and quick to grow and supplied good nourishment. Later in World War II the roots gained more recognition in a number of countries as they could be purchased without ration cards. Lewis and Clark, the famous explorers, used Jerusalem artichokes for sustenance during their expedition when food was difficult to come by.

Health Benefits of Jerusalem artichokes

Jerusalem artichokes provide a number of health benefits due to the nutrients found in them. They are high in potassium, an element necessary for maintenance of overall health. It is beneficial for individuals at risk of elevated blood pressure levels. Consumption of the vegetable on a regular basis can help to maintain healthy blood cholesterol level which is essential for your heart health. Just one cup of the root delivers 25% of the daily iron needs. To get the same amount from red meat you would have to consume three ounces of it! Iron is a necessary component of the red blood cells, needed to deliver oxygen to all parts of the body. Deficiency of the element results in fatigue and lowered immunity. Sun-chokes are loaded with protein. It has especially high quantities of sulphur containing amino acids taurine, methionine, homocysteine and cysteine. These compounds are necessary for connective tissue flexibility along with detoxification of the body.

Additional benefits include:

- Low calories make it a good addition to any weight loss program.
- Aids in standardizing metabolism.
- Being rich in inulin and dietary fibre makes them good for diabetics.

- Alleviates constipation.
- Rids the body of toxins.
- Provides strength to the immune system.

Nutritional Value Jerusalem artichokes

Jerusalem artichokes are highly nutritious tubers. A one cup serving of raw artichoke contains only 110 calories, approximately 26 grams of carbohydrates, three grams of protein, and ten grams of fibre. This translates to 10% of the daily fibre needs, 9% of the carbohydrate needs and 6% of the required amount of protein. Better yet they contain almost no fat, sodium or saturated fat and cholesterol.

Jerusalem artichokes are heavily fortified with vitamins as well. Just one serving of the veggie provides 28% of the recommended daily allowance of iron, 14% potassium, 9% phosphorous and 6% magnesium. Additionally it supplies 25% of thiamine, 12% niacin, 7% riboflavin and vitamin C and 5% of folate and vitamin B12.

Uses of Jerusalem artichokes

Much of the sun chokes' nutrients are found immediately below the skin and peeling the tuber means wasting a lot of the nutrients. It is best to scrub the tuber with a vegetable brush. Sun chokes discolour rapidly upon cutting, so make sure to cut them very close to serving time. If it is necessary to prepare them in advance, then cut them and submerge them in water with added lemon juice or a couple to tablespoons of vinegar. This will prevent oxidation and maintain the colour. When cooked in the skin, it turns a dark colour due to the large amounts of iron.

Jerusalem artichokes have no downside, which makes them the ideal addition to many foods or used on their own. They can be sprinkled in sandwiches, salads and as garnish in soups. They can be served with dips, shredded into coleslaw, marinated in lemon juice or rice vinegar. They can be used to make soups.

A few more serving ideas:

- They can be used in stir fries along with other vegetables in olive oil. To get a crisp texture, fry for only two to four minutes, for softer texture fry a little longer.
- You can slice the artichokes and drizzle them with a little olive oil, then place them on a cookie sheet to bake at 375 degrees for approximately 25 minutes. Alternatively, you can bake the whole tuber like a potato.
- To steam the veggie just chop and place it in a streamer, cover and allow to cook for roughly 6 to 8 minutes. They can be enjoyed by seasoning to taste or they can be mashed like potatoes.

By far one of the best ways to enjoy Jerusalem artichokes is to juice them or add them to smoothies. Here are a couple of recipes that are sure to not only quench thirst but leave you invigorated.

Zesty Sun-choke Juice
- 2 stalks celery
- ½ cup sun-chokes
- ½ cucumber
- ½ teaspoon lemon juice

Juice and drink chilled.

Sweet & Spicy Sun-choke Smoothie
- 1 small apple or (½ of a large one)
- 1 ½ chopped carrot
- ½ cup chopped sun-choke
- 1 clove garlic
- ¼ inch ginger
- Fist full of cilantro and parsley

Place all ingredients in a blender and thoroughly blend.

Clinical Trials

High blood pressure is a major precursor to cardiovascular disease. Although the market is full of synthesized drugs, each comes with its own set of side effects, leading to a search for natural remedies for the treatment or prevention of the ailment. Prebiotics from dietary sources is considered a possible acceptable alternative. Prebiotics are food particles that cannot be digested and by sidestepping digestion they reach the large intestine as food for resident good bacteria. Studies show that these prebiotics have the potential to cut down and prevent hypertension[1].

Sun-chokes are loaded with the compound inulin. This non-digestible fibre has prebiotic characteristics. When fermentation of this compound takes place, the derivatives produced block the growth of cancerous tumour cells in the colon[2].

Resources

[1]http://www.ncbi.nlm.nih.gov/pubmed/20111692

[2] http://www.ncbi.nlm.nih.gov/pubmed/15877900

Kale

Introduction to Kale

Kale (*Brassica oleracea*), also sometimes referred to as borecole, is a relative of the more highly developed members of the same family like broccoli, cauliflower and Brussels sprouts. The vegetable has been so popular in Scotland that "come to kale" was an invitation to dinner. In addition to the typical green colour the vegetable is available in white, purple and pink too!

Kale is essentially a primitive cabbage that has held on to its characteristics since prehistoric times. The reason for kale's perseverance is due to its virtues as a garden vegetable. Different varieties of kale are cultivated all around the world and while it grows well in various climates, it does particularly well in the cooler winter months. In fact some people claim their taste is sweeter when harvested after the first frost. While a member of the cabbage family, kale does not have a head, instead there are long fibrous stalks cascading outward from a centre bunch.

During World War II, kale was cultivated widely due to ease of growing and it supplemented the meagre war time rationing while supplying important nutrients. Once the war was finished, a lot of families moved away from kale, due to the association of its taste, and texture with wartime deprivations.

History of Kale

Kale is the descendent of the wild cabbage which has its origins in Asia Minor. Kale is a member of the *Acephala* cultivar, hence the full name *Brassica oleracea acephala* translates to "cabbage of the vegetable garden without a head". The ruffled look of its leaves differentiate it from the more smooth leafed collard greens of the same family.

Kale was introduced to Europe by Celtic explorers around 600 B.C.E, and prevailed on the continent for over 2000 years. It was among the most common green vegetable until the middle ages when cabbage started to gain acceptance. Kale played a vital role in early European food supplies and was a major crop in the ancient Roman era, known to Romans by the name of Sabelline Cabbage. Its high yield and ease of cultivation made it a popular vegetable among the peasants during the Middle Ages. Almost every Scottish household grew kale in their yards, known as "kaleyards", due to its hardiness and they preserved it in barrels of salt. If a Scot was "off his kale", it meant he was too ill to eat. Kale holds a vital position in cuisine of Scandinavia and Holland, and in Germany, "Kale King" is crowned during the annual kale festival. English settlers carried kale to the New World in the 17th century.

The Japanese bred the very first varieties of ornamental kale we see today. They first appeared in seed catalogs in the 1930s. The central leaves of ornamental varieties may be pink, rose, violet, yellow or white to creamy in colour, while the outer leaves are varying shades of green, blue or gray. The wrinkly edges give a ruffled ornate effect. The colour of the leaf becomes more intense after the first frost. While it is essentially a decorative plant, it can quiet easily be eaten also. The only difference between the decoration kale and the green kale is the pigmentation in leaves. The pigmentation has no affect on the taste of the leaf, but ornamental varieties are hardly ever sold for consumption mainly due to the high expense associated with them.

Health Benefits of Kale

Kale contains at least forty five flavonoids, and a wide array of vitamins and minerals. It offers benefits in three main areas: The high anti-inflammatory and antioxidant nutrients, the micronutrients a body requires in small quantities but can't produce itself, and the cancer protecting glucosinolates (compounds housing sulphur and nitrogen that incite the body's antioxidant system into action).

Kale is a low calorie food which is high in fibre content. This makes it the ideal food for individuals trying to lose weight, and the fibre helps in digestion and keeps movement of waste from the body steady. It provides more iron per calorie than beef and iron benefits the system by aiding in proper liver function, transportation of oxygen to all parts of the body and during formation of haemoglobin and enzymes. The high vitamin K content helps in keeping bones healthy, preventing blood clotting and elevated vitamin K levels also help people with Alzheimer's disease. Antioxidants such as flavonoids and carotenoids offer protection against a number of cancers. The anti-inflammatory compound omega-3 fatty acids fight off arthritis, asthma and autoimmune ailments. Kale is also known to help stabilize cholesterol levels. The vitamin A in kale helps with vision, skin and lung cancer while vitamin C keeps metabolism in check and enhances the immune system. Kale has more calcium per calorie than milk, which prevents bone loss, osteoporosis and aids in maintaining healthy metabolism. The phytonutrients like quercetin prevent plaque formation, thus keeping the circulatory system healthy.

While kale is considered to be a very healthy food, excessive amounts can interfere with certain drugs like anticoagulants. It is associated with haemolytic anemia, where red blood cells breakdown to the point of threatening life. It is also high in oxalates that can interfere with calcium absorption. This simply means you should not be drinking a litre of kale in smoothies every day. You are now aware of the issues and should use it in moderation so you can benefit from its good points without being affected by its weak points.

Nutritional Value of Kale

In recent years kale has come to be known as one of the "superfoods", and even cooked it delivers loads of vitamins and minerals. It is low in calories delivering only 28 in a 100 gram serving, and fat with only 0.4 grams. At the same time it provides 1.9 grams of protein and 2 grams of fibre. Out of the 100 gram serving 91.2 grams are water and 5.63 grams carbohydrates.

A one hundred gram serving of kale provides 778% of vitamin K, 85% of vitamin A, 49% vitamin C, 11% vitamin B6, 6% vitamin B2 and E, 5% vitamin B1, and 3% vitamin B3 and B9. Kale is rich in mineral content also, with a single one hundred gram serving delivering 20% manganese, 7% each of iron and calcium, 5% magnesium and potassium, 4% phosphorus, 3% zinc, and 2% zinc.

Uses of Kale

Kale is very fibrous so most people prefer to eat it cooked instead of consuming it raw. In either case, the woody stem needs to be removed before using kale.

Kale can be steamed, boiled, sautéed, baked or stir fried. Kale makes a good addition to stews and soups as its hardy leaves hold up well even when boiled. Kale can be added to salads using an oil based dressing which helps in softening the stiff leaves. The slightly bitter taste of raw kale makes a nice contrast to things like honey and tahini.

In the U.S kale is typically used in combination with other greens like turnip leaves and collard. It is braised for hours with ham hock. It is also well accepted as a smoothie ingredient, due to its high nutritional value and fibre content. Baking it until turns it into a crunchy "chip" providing a healthy alternative to the potato chip.

Creamy Kale Smoothie
- 1 cup frozen strawberries
- 1 cup frozen cherries
- ½ cup apple juice
- 2 leaves of kale
- ¼ tsp. cinnamon powder
- 1 tbsp, yogurt

Instructions: Put everything into a blender and puree until smooth.

Clinical Trials

A fairly new study published in the Journal of Nutrition (2004) found that sulforaphane found in kale helps to halt proliferation of breast cancer cells. Sulforaphane forms when kale is cut up or chewed. This compound makes the liver produce natural enzymes that go on to detoxify cancer forming chemicals from our bodies[1, 2].

In another study of lung cancer patients, it was found that elevated consumption of cruciferous vegetables like kale reduced lung cancer risk by 39%[2].

According to some studies, sulforaphane encourages a healthy immune system which in turn averts cancer. It increased the production of a number of chemicals that take part in the immune response[3].

Sulforaphane also has a direct effect on colon cancer. In one study, genetically bred animals that developed intestinal polyps, a precursor to tumour formation, were fed sulforaphane. The group of animals fed sulforaphane were found to have enhanced rates of cell suicide and smaller tumours developed more slowly as compared to animals that were not given sulforaphane[4].

Kale is rich in carotenoids, plant pigments known to absorb blue light. Two carotenoids kale is especially endowed with are lutein and zeaxanthin, and both of them behave like filters that avert eye damage from exposure to ultraviolet light. In a number of studies people who consume kale like lutein-rich foods had 22% reduced risk of cancer[5].

Lutein also aids in averting artherosclerosis. According to an 18 month long study at University of Southern California, people with minimum serum lutein concentration had five times higher carotid artery thickness, an indicator of heart disease risk, compared to people who had greatest serum lutein concentrations. Additionally it was found that cells pre-treated with lutein protected them against inflammation linked with LDL plaque development. This again proved that lutein offers protections against arterosclerosis[6].

Resources

[1] http://whatscookingamerica.net/LindaPosch/Kale.htm

[2] Wang LI, Giovannucci EL, Hunter D, Neuberg D, Su L, Christiani DC. Dietary intake of Cruciferous vegetables, Glutathione S-transferase (GST) polymorphisms and lung cancer risk in a Caucasian population. Cancer Causes Control. Dec 2004;15(10):977-85.

[3]Thejass P, Kuttan G. Augmentation of natural killer cell and antibody-dependent cellular cytotoxicity in BALB/c mice by sulforaphane, a naturally occurring isothiocyanate from broccoli through enhanced production of cytokines IL-2 and IFN-gamma. Immunopharmacol Immunotoxicol. 2006;28(3):443-57.

[4] Khor TO, Hu R, Shen G, et al. Pharmacogenomics of cancer chemopreventive isothiocyanate compound sulforaphane in the intestinal polyps of ApcMin/+ mice. Biopharm Drug Dispos. Dec 2006;27(9):407-20.

[5] Brown L, Rimm EB, Seddon JM, et al. A prospective study of carotenoid intake and risk of cataract extraction in US men. Am J Clin Nutr. Oct 1999;70(4):517-24.

[6] Dwyer JH, Navab M, Dwyer KM, et al. Oxygenated carotenoid lutein and progression of early atherosclerosis: the Los Angeles atherosclerosis study. Circulation. 2001 Jun 19;103(24):2922-7.

Kiwifruit

Introduction Kiwifruit

The kiwifruit is also known by its short name, kiwi, in some parts of the world as well as Chinese gooseberry, and Yang Tao. Interior of the fruit is dazzling green flesh with radiating lighter green spikes. Scattered between the spikes are the miniature edible dark purple to almost black seeds. The flesh is soft and juicy with a creamy texture and sweet/tart (at times acidic) flavour. Exterior is a brown coloured skin covered by short, stiff, dense hairs.

Actinidia deliciosa (kiwi) is actually a berry capable of growing anywhere citrus fruits can grow. The plant is able to lie dormant in sub-zero temperatures, after which it flourishes and produces flowers of cream colour roughly one to two inches in size. Both male and female flowers have to be present for the female to be able to produce the fruit. However, one male plant is able to pollinate many female plants. The pollination in carried out by the typical garden animals like honey bees and butterflies, or even the wind.

History of Kiwifruit

Originating in the Yangtze Valley of northern China, the kiwifruit is known to have been cultivated for at least three hundred years. The Chinese never showed much interest in exploiting the fruit, nor expanding its local cultivation initially. It was grown in an area of dense population and growth was restricted.

In 1900 seeds made their way into England, where the plants bloomed and flourished by 1909. While fruits were produced where male and female plants existed side by side, for the most parts only solitary vines were planted for ornamental purposes. At about this time, seeds were also introduced to New Zealand with the vines producing fruit by 1910. By the 1930s different people were propagating the plants. As production grew so did the marketing and the fruit became very popular with the American servicemen based in New Zealand in World War II. By 1953 commercial export to Japan, North America and Europe and to a lesser degree to Australia, U.K and Scandinavia started. In

1962 the increasing demand, and to further increase its market appeal, the name of the fruit was officially changed from Chinese gooseberry to kiwifruit. This name was chosen as a tribute to the native New Zealand kiwi bird whose physical characteristics of fuzzy brown coat are similar to kiwifruit's skin. New Zealand was responsible for supplying 99% of kiwifruit's global requirement.

From New Zealand the plants and seeds ended up in the U.S.A. with special nurseries taking root in 1966. The Fruit and Fruit Technology Research Institute of Stellenbosch, South Africa also started experimental plantings in different places in the country. The vines grew with success in north-eastern Transvaal. The fruit was already being cultivated in Cambodia, Vietnam, Laos, France, Spain, Belgium and Italy. With lower returns from apple growing, French interest was rejuvenated in kiwi production in 1971. Greece stepped up production for export to Europe to cover the seasonal gap when New Zealand fruit was not available. Currently, Italy, New Zealand, Chile, France, Japan and the United States are the world's top producers of kiwis.

Health Benefits of Kiwifruit

While the Chinese have never favoured the fruit, even they have used it as a tonic for children during the growing years and women after child birth. Recent popularity of the fruit has only intensified the research into its beneficial properties and according to the University of Innsbruck, Austria, consuming a fruit that is ripe to the point of spoiling only enhances the beneficial aspects of the fruit.

Kiwis contain a naturally high quantity of antioxidants and other phytochemicals that help to enhance the immune system function by fighting off stress, inflammation and bacterial and viral attacks. The high fibre content adds roughage and the proteolytic enzyme actinidin facilitates the digestion of proteins for smooth flow of food through the digestive tract at an even pace. The polysaccharides in Kiwis prevent the bonding of enteropathogens and trigger the probiotic bacteria in the colon into action. The steady movement of food through the digestive tract also regulates blood sugar absorption which eliminates undesirable sugar spikes and troughs, making it an ideal fruit for diabetics. Furthermore, consuming a diet high in fibre is believed to lower cholesterol levels which in turn protects against heart disease.

The elevated vitamin C content in the fruit rids the body of free radicals known to damage healthy cells. This helps to cut down on the inflammation in bone and connective tissues and alleviating symptoms of rheumatoid arthritis or osteoarthritis. Elimination of free radicals is also associated with protection against various cancers like lung, colon, mouth, and stomach. Kiwifruit is cytotoxic to malignant cancer cells and does not harm the healthy cells. Catechin, a phytochemical found in kiwi reduces the toxicity and stimulates bone marrow production. Vitamin C is also associated with lowering blood pressure by properly dilating blood vessels and preventing problems like atherosclerosis, cholesterol and cardiovascular disease. It is also believed to reduce the triglycerides in the blood, thus helping to prevent blood clots. Kiwi fruit has more vitamin C than oranges and benefits the respiratory system against ailments like asthma, cough and shortness of breath.

The phytochemicals lutein and zeaxanthin found in kiwi benefit eye health. These components are essential to the human eye along with vitamin A and protect against age-linked macular degeneration, cataracts and other vision disorders. The folate in kiwis is essential for protecting the unborn baby from neural tube defects and contributes to the overall health of the developing foetus.

Kiwis are natural anti-aging agents. The vitamin E in kiwi helps to eliminate the fine lines thus reducing wrinkles, in addition to minimizing the effects of ultra-violet radiation on the skin. The vitamin C keeps the skin firm and speeds up the process of healing in case of cuts and abrasions. Kiwis also aids in collagen synthesis which keeps the skin smooth and retain it natural elasticity leading to younger looking skin.

Nutritional Value of Kiwifruit

Kiwifruit is rich in nutrients but low in calories. One cup of sliced kiwifruit supplies 5 grams (16 % of the U.S Recommended Daily Allowance) of fibre to help keep your digestive system in top shape. It supplies both soluble fibre that plays a protective role in heart disease and insoluble fibre responsible for averting problems like constipation, and haemorrhoids.

There are few other foods that provide equivalent amounts of folic acid as kiwi. Folate is such an essential vitamin that several countries are thinking of adding it to bread or flour to make certain that the population gets sufficient quantities. While bananas are often thought of as a good source of potassium, kiwifruit supplies roughly the same amount without the calories. Kiwi is the perfect low sodium way to get sufficient quantities of potassium. One serving of kiwi has 20% more potassium than a banana. Oranges have a long established reputation of being a good source of vitamin C, but kiwis have even more. One serving provides roughly 230% of the U.S Recommended Daily Allowance. It also supplies 10% of the RDA of vitamin E, which is twice as much as that of an avocado.

Kiwi is ranked higher than all other fruits and veggies, except yellow corn for lutein. It also supplies 5.5% of the RDA of calcium, 4% iron, 6% magnesium and 8% copper. It provides trace amounts of manganese required by enzymes in protein metabolism and food energy, and chromium, a key element in regulation of heartbeat and carbohydrate metabolism.

Uses of Kiwifruit

Kiwifruit's characteristic looks and rejuvenating taste make them great to eat fresh. They can easily be peeled with a paring knife and enjoyed sliced or they may be cut in half and the flesh scooped out with a spoon. The skin too is edible like that of a pear and only enhances the nutrients and fibre of the fruit. The fuzzy hairs can be easily rubbed off before consumption. Kiwi should be eaten soon after cutting as the enzymes actinic and bromic acids have food tenderizing properties and tend to tenderize the fruit itself.

Kiwi can be served as an appetizer, in salads, fowl, meat dishes, salads, pies, puddings, cake-fillings and with ice-cream, breads and as a variety of beverages. When serving in salads it is best to put kiwi in at the last moment so it doesn't make the salad soggy. Likewise it is best not to use kiwifruit with yogurt and gelatin-based products because the enzymes present in it break down the proteins in these foods. If it has to be used with these products, then cook the fruit for a few minutes to neutralize the enzymes. These very same properties make kiwi a great meat tenderizer. Simply rub the meat with the kiwi flesh, or place slices of kiwifruit on the meat. Remove or scrape off the fruit after about ten minutes or the enzymatic action can be extreme. For best results, cook the meat immediately.

The over ripe fruits are used as flavours in ice cream and for commercial production of juice. It is typically blended with apples to minimize the acidity. The under-ripe fruits are selected for turning into jelly, jam and chutney. Freeze dried fruits are sold in health food outlets in Sweden and Japan. In Japan they are even sold coated with chocolate. Whole fruits are also good to pickle with vinegar, brown sugar and spices.

Clinical Trials

Numerous clinical trials investigating various health benefits of kiwifruit are being investigated in different laboratories. The vitamin C in kiwi is linked to protection against asthma. One study published in April 2004 issue of Thorax found children consuming more kiwifruit had 44% fewer incidences of wheezing[1].

According to another study, the serotonin in kiwifruit aids in sleeping better. Consumption of the fruit helped with total sleep time and efficiency. The flavonoids quercitin, catechin, rutin, naringenin and epicatechin modulate sleep generating receptors, working as a sedative. Kiwi peel is a powerful ingredient for developing natural sleeping aids[2].

Another astounding benefit of kiwifruit is its capability to accommodate absorption of iron by the body. The phytochemicals lutein and zeaxanthin found in kiwi improve the presence of iron in the body and prevent iron deficiency ailments[3]. In another study it was shown that kiwi helps to regulate adipogenesis, which is vital in diabetes prevention[4].

Resources

[1]http://kiwifruit.org/media/did-you-know.aspx

[2]http://www.ncbi.nlm.nih.gov/pubmed/21669584

[3]http://www.ncbi.nlm.nih.gov/pubmed/20727238

[4]http://www.ncbi.nlm.nih.gov/pubmed/20087882

Lemon

A member of the Rutaceae family, the botanical name of a lemon is Citrus Limonum. The true lemon tree reaches a height of 10 to 20 feet (three to six meters), and is full of twigs with sharp thorns. The flowers with their mild fragrance can be clustered or solitary, and are white in colour with purplish undersides. Once open, the followers yield four to five petals. The fruit is technically a berry (hesperidium), and can range in size from 2 ¾ inches to 4 ¾ in with the number of seeds inside varying according to variety. The juice of a lemon is 5% to 6% citric acid, giving them their sour taste. Lemon peel is usually of light yellow colouration, although some varieties may be dappled with long green stripes. The peel is aromatic and houses oil glands ranging ¼ to ⅜ inch (6-10 mm) in thickness.

There are three basic types of lemon. The most widely available is the acidic kind, which is easily obtainable at supermarkets. Then there are the primitive lemons used to propagate different types of citrus fruits like oranges and limes. Finally there are the sweet lemons, once a mere curiosity, but now slowly gaining popularity with the development of the Meyer lemon.

Lemons lend themselves well to medicinal and culinary purposes. Lemon juice is a formidable and pleasant antiseptic. Traditionally, the major medicinal use of lemons has been for scurvy or to relieve vomiting. It the past, lemon juice was also employed to alleviate rheumatic fever, gout and rheumatism. Lemon drops were one of the very first candies ever produced. They were made by boiling down a mixture of sugar and lemon juice, and then pouring the mix into sheet moulds. Once firm, the sheets were simply dropped to shatter the candy into separate pieces.

History of Lemon

The Lemon is said to have originated somewhere in the Indus Valley. This is based on archaeological evidence, among which are lemon-shaped earring dating back to 2500 BCE. Arab traders are credited with bringing lemons to the Middle East and Africa around 100 BCE. From there it was launched into southern Italy around 200 BCE. The lemon was valued for its medicinal properties in the palaces of Sultan of Egypt and Syria. While rare and costly, lemons can even be seen in a mosaic in Pompeii.

Initially, lemons were more of an ornamental plant, like tomatoes, rather than a source of food. They were used to give red colour to lips by the ladies at King Louis XIV's court. Cesare Borgia sent lemons as presents to his bride in France, and to flaunt his wealth in front of Louis XII. In the eleventh century, lemons were introduced to Spain by the Arabs, and by 1150 they were a commonly cultivated crop in the Mediterranean. Crusaders going home from Palestine introduced them all over Europe, and lemons gained popularity when cookbooks started to recommend replacing the existing traditions of extreme spiciness with juice from lemons.

It wasn't until the 15th century that full gastronomic use of lemons started in Europe. The first significant cultivation was in Genoa. Lemons travelled to the New World in 1493 with Christopher Columbus taking the seeds to Hispaniola. While the Spanish conquest helped in proliferating lemons throughout the area, they were still mainly used for ornamental and medicinal purposes. By 1751 lemon cultivation had started in California and by the 1800s in Florida, when their use for culinary purposes picked up.

The origins of the word "lemon" lie in the Middle English word *limon,* and it first surfaced around the middle to end of the fourteenth century. Limon is actually an Old French word, which shows that lemon came to England through France. Old French has its beginnings in Italian *limone,* which comes from the Arabic word *laymun* derived from the Persian limun.

Guatemala and Mexico are among the major lemon producers. Their primary purpose is to extract the oil out of the peel, and the secondary purpose is to dehydrate the juice for preparation of reconstituted juice. Argentina leads the lemon production in South America, while Italy, Spain, Greece, Cyprus, Turkey, Lebanon, Australia, and South Africa are the world's foremost lemon producers.

Health Benefits Associated with Lemon

Lemon is beneficial for a wide variety of ailments. In Italy, sweetened lemon juice is used to alleviate stomatitis, gingivitis, and inflammation of the tongue. A drink of warm water and lemon is advocated as a laxative, and it's also believed to avert the common cold. Warm lemon water is offered in some of the most exclusive spas. Lemon juice with honey or ginger is frequently used as a cold remedy. It is a diuretic (for water loss), anti-scorbutic (scurvy), an astringent (something that draws tissue together), and a febrifuge (to reduce fever). Lemon juice was used by sailors aboard British ships in the 18th Century to help counter scurvy where they became known as "limeys".

Vitamin C found is found in abundant supply within lemons and acts as a potent antioxidant. As it passes through the body, it neutralizes free radicals that come into its path. Free radicals interfere with healthy cells to render them useless, thus leading to aging, inflammation, and other ailments. Vitamin C also helps to provide relief from respiratory and breathing problems like asthma.

Being a natural antiseptic, lemon juice spread over the skin can reduce pain caused by sun burn and bee stings. The fruit is also used to treat acne, and eczema. It can behave as an anti-aging solution by removing wrinkles and blackheads. Applying lemon juice on old burns can help to fade scars. Its coagulating properties can help to stop internal bleeding while cotton soaked in lemon juice can help to stop nose bleeds. Being a diuretic, it helps to remove toxins from the body thus aiding people suffering from illnesses like cholera and malaria.

Applying lemon juice to the hair and scalp provide a natural shine to the hair and also helps to eliminate problems like dandruff, and hair loss. Lemon applied to an aching tooth can help to get rid of the pain, and massaging it on gums puts a stop to gum bleeds and bad breath.

More recent claims on the benefits of lemon state that it is a miracle product that is ten thousand times stronger than chemotherapy with the ability to fight off many types of cancers. However, pharmaceutical laboratories interested in creating synthetic versions and pocketing profits do not publicize the fact[1].

While this claim may be a bit excessive, lemons do provide many benefits. In a study carried out by Foschi R., Pelucchi C., Dal Maso L., et al., it was found that the chances of developing stomach, throat, mouth, colon, and lung airways cancer was markedly less in individuals with a high intake of lemons, but there was no effect on breast, endometrial, kidney, ovarian and prostate cancers[2].

Furthermore, lemons are packed with a variety of phytochemicals like Hesperetin, limonene, naringin, and naringenin. It is the naringenin which is responsible for scavenging free radicals and providing the anti-inflammatory, antioxidant properties. Minute quantities of vitamin A, and flavonoids like α, and ß-carotenes, ß-cryptoxanthin, zeaxanthin and lutein are also found in lemons.

The Many Uses of Lemon

Lemons provide a tangy and refreshing flavour to both sweet and savoury dishes, in addition to being good cleaning and refreshing agents. Sprinkled on vegetables, salads, soups, rice, sushi, and to perk up drinks, the list of culinary uses is endless. Both the juice and peel of the lemon can be used. Here are some other unconventional uses of this citrus fruit:

- Lemon juice is great for brightening up yellowed nails. Squeeze a lemon in a dish and soak your nails in the juice for a few minutes.
- Applying lemon juice to fruits and vegetables like potatoes, pears, apples, and avocados, prevents them from going brown. Droopy lettuce can be brought back to life by soaking it in a bowl of cold water with the juice of one lemon squeezed into it.
- Run out of deodorant? Just cut a lemon in half and apply under your arms. The citric acid kills odour producing bacteria and keeps you fresh.
- Lemons are great as insect deterrents. Bugs like spiders, fleas, ants and even cockroaches are sensitive to the smell. Squirting lemon juice in places where they may enter the house will keep them at bay. Better yet, add a little lemon to your floor wash for greater insect-repelling power.

- Lemon juice eliminates hard water stains, and other stubborn marks. For tough stains, use straight or dilute and use out of a spray bottle. Lemon is also great for sparkling transparent windows.
- Mildew, berries, wine or oil, in fact almost all substances that can leave stains on fabric can be gotten rid of with lemon juice. Tougher fabrics can be rubbed with lemon juice and salt, while more delicate fabrics may require a more gentle treatment.

No part of the lemon should be wasted because the peel of a lemon contains five to ten times more nutrients than the juice. To utilize the whole fruit, just put it in the freezer overnight and freeze it. Once frozen, grate the solidified lemon and discard only the pits. The rest of the lemon may be used to sprinkle as garnish on top of any food desired.

Clinical Trials

There are a number of studies reporting on the medicinal value of lemons. A 2002 report by the University of Florida's Institute of Food and Agricultural Sciences, states that compounds like flavanoids, carotenoids, and limonoids have potential antiviral, anti-cancer, and anti-inflammatory properties. Additionally they have the ability to lower cholesterol[1].

Another study published by the Texas A&M University's Kingsville Citrus Centre, states that limonoids found in lemons seek out neuroblastomas and stops them. Neuroblastomas are responsible for ten percent of all child cancers[3].

Resources

[1] http://www.snopes.com/medical/disease/lemons.asp

[2] Foschi R., Pelucchi C., Dal Maso L., Et al. Cancer Causes Control. 2010 Feb; 21 (2): 237-42

[3] http://www.sciencedaily.com/releases/2004/11/041130203424.htm

Lettuce

Lettuce is the type of a vegetable that just about all plant breeders like to meddle with, hence the seemingly endless varieties! Ranging in colour anywhere from crispy green to crimson red, the flavours and nutritional values of the different varieties also vary greatly. Lettuce belongs to the Asteraceae family with the scientific name Lactuca sativa. With small annual plants, the leaves of Lactuca sativa excrete milk like liquid (sap) upon cutting. The name lactuca (lac meaning milk) is derived from Latin. Lettuce can be grouped into seven basic types with numerous sub-varieties in each. They are distinguished from one another based on formation of their heads and leaves. The leaf varieties tend to be a little bitter, but loaded with antioxidants. The main lettuce types are as follows:

Loose-leaf lettuces are generally multi-coloured, delicate with well flavoured leaves, and are a fast growing variety. They form loose open heads which makes it convenient to harvest just a few leaves or the whole head according to needs.

Butterhead lettuces are another group with open loose leaves and have a buttery texture. This variety is more popular in Europe.

Romaine (Cos) are upright, tall, and have open heads with deep green coloured leaves. The leaves carry a stronger flavour compared to the loose-leaf variety, and contain a prominent crunchy midrib that travels all the way to the tip of the leaf.

Buttercrunch lettuces are a cross between romaine and the butterhead varieties. The head has a more upright stature than romaine, with hardly any leaves touching the ground. This group is better able to withstand the cold weather than butterhead, with leaves that defy rotting.

Batavian Lettuces have crunchy, thick leaves. The leaves of Batavian Lettuces can tolerate heat better than all other varieties.

Heading lettuces curl their leaves inward forming heads similar to those of cabbages. These are the basic iceberg lettuces valued for their ability to resist disease and heat. They have a solid watery crunch and very little flavour or nutritional value.

Chinese lettuces are strong flavoured with rather stiff, long, non-head forming leaves. They are valued not only for their leaves but the stalks as well. They are slightly bitter in taste, but do well in soups and stir-fries.

History of Lettuce

Egyptians started the cultivation of lettuce from a weed at least 4500 BC, the seeds of which were used to produce oil. Depictions of lettuce can be seen in Egyptian tombs. The Egyptians used lettuce as fertility medicine. It spread to the Greeks and Romans, and both cultures valued it highly, both as a food and for its medicinal properties. The Romans named it 'lactuca', which eventually lead to the English 'lettuce'.

Several varieties of lettuce were known by 50 AD, and it was frequently named in medieval writings. From the 16th to 18th centuries, many additional varieties were developed in Europe. In the medieval era, it was believed that lettuce possessed medicinal qualities, and was prescribed for a number of diseases. It was used to cure appetite loss, blood pressure irregularity, as a tonic for the digestive system, and to limit sexual urges. Dried lettuce latex was prescribed as a cure for insomnia, as nasal drops, as an antispasmodic, and a sedative.

Lettuce had been grown in China as early as the 5th century. To the Chinese, lettuce represents good luck and is served on special occasions like birthdays, weddings and New Year's Day, etc. Christopher Columbus is credited with introducing lettuce to North America in 1493 during his second voyage. By the nineteenth century, the use of lettuce had spread to the rest of world. Today this leaf vegetable can be found in literally every corner of the planet.

Health Benefits of the Lettuce

Regular consumption of lettuce is believed to have numerous health benefits. It has dietary fibre and Omega fatty acids, both of which are important for general health. The roughage helps to enhance bulk in the intestines, thereby improving peristalsis and eliminating constipation and other stomach problems.

Additionally, the high folate content is good for maintaining cardiovascular health and for putting off arteriosclerosis and stroke. Minerals like potassium, phosphorus, and manganese, destroy free radicals which damage cells, improve immune system function, and offer protection against viral infections. The iron in lettuce aids in the transport of oxygen for cell growth and blood distribution within the body. This makes lettuce the ideal food for anaemic patients. It is also helpful for insomniacs as it contains substances that induce sleep.

It is said that the regular consumption of lettuce juice helps to improve the rate of fertility, raises sperm count, and also helps with erectile dysfunction and early ejaculation issues. Furthermore, it is believed to put a stop to habitual miscarriages and has an effect on progesterone release, something which is liable for lactation in mothers who are breast feeding.

Nutritional Value

Of the different varieties of lettuce available in the market, the three types that are most favoured include, leaf, head, and romaine (cos). Other types also have varying kinds and amounts of nutrients. The Romaine lettuce is considered the most nutrient rich among all the varieties, while iceberg lettuce has the least nutritional value.

Iceberg lettuce has almost no cholesterol and very little fat. It is abundant in dietary fibre and folate, has some fatty acids, and trace amounts of omega fatty acids. It has lower amounts of vitamin C, A, iron, potassium, phosphorous, zinc, sodium, magnesium, manganese, calcium and amino acids than its dark green leaved cousins.

Romaine lettuce is a good source of Vitamins B6, E, A, K, and C. It supplies some dietary fibre through its ribs and spine, carbohydrates, and protein. Additionally, it contains the minerals, calcium, iron, magnesium, phosphorous, potassium, sodium, zinc (along with thiamin), riboflavin, niacin, and folate. It also naturally concentrates and absorbs lithium.

How to Use Lettuce

The best lettuce is purchased fresh and should have, crisp leaves that are devoid of dark or slimy spots. The best way to use lettuce is to ensure it is garden fresh, discard any tarnished leaves, chop to desired size, and throw away the lower stem. Wash the leaves under cold running water and then let soak in salt water for approximately ½ an hour to get rid of sand and any parasite worms and eggs. Finally pat dry before use.

Some serving ideas:

- Fresh, uncooked lettuce may be used in sandwiches, burgers, salads or spring rolls.
- It may be stir fried, stewed, and supplement noodles or fried rice.
- It can be combined with seafood, green beans, and peas.

Traditional Use Methods

Traditionally, the Romans consumed their lettuce with an oil and vinegar dressing, while the lettuce with smaller leaves was just eaten raw. During the reign of Domitian (81 – 96 AD), the concept of serving lettuce before a meal started. In Europe, after the Roman rule, the tradition of poaching lettuce continued, especially with the romaine variety.

Little Lettuce Enfolds

This is a really nice alternative to the typical family meal. It is not only nutritious, but also something that kids really enjoy. It allows you to make alterations according to your tastes. In the recipe below I am using chicken, but there is no reason why you can substitute this with beef, tuna, or turkey.

Ingredients:

- ½ pound of ground chicken
- ½ cup of water chestnuts, chopped
- ½ cup of mushrooms, chopped
- 1 small carrot, chopped

- 1½ tablespoon of soy sauce
- ½ tablespoon of oyster sauce
- ½ teaspoon of ginger
- Salt and pepper to taste
- 1-2 cloves of garlic, crushed
- ½ tablespoon of olive oil
- Iceberg lettuce, separated leaves

Directions:

In a small bowl, combine soy sauce, oyster sauce, and ginger, then place aside.

Heat olive oil over a medium heat in a large skillet. Add the chicken and stir-fry, breaking it up while cooking. When about half cooked, add the vegetables to the chicken, along with chestnuts and the sauce mixture. Continue to cook until most of the liquid disappears. Season with salt and pepper to taste (the sauce mixture is fairly salty, so take care with the salt!).

For serving; spoon the meat mixture onto the middle of the lettuce leaf, and wrap the lettuce around it making a cylindrical shaped rod.

Clinical Trials

As reported in the "Journal of Young Investigators" back in August 2007, The University of Central Florida cultivated genetically modified lettuce that has the potential to treat insulin dependent diabetics. The lettuce was able to cure diabetes in mice, but human trials are still inconclusive. The special genetically altered lettuce manufactures insulin that is housed in the plant's chloroplast cells, and is not damaged by the stomach's acid. The intestinal bacteria helps to release the insulin which then makes its way into the bloodstream to remove excessive glucose.[1]

Wild lettuce has shown to have benefits for anxiety and anxiety related disorders. Some subjective evidence suggests that lettuce may relieve insomnia, a key anxiety disorder. The "Journal of Clinical Sleep Medicine" published a clinical review in 2005 of the use of lettuce for insomnia. The lactucin, a component of wild lettuce, generated pain-eliminating and sedative like effects, according to another study published in the September 2006 issue of "Journal of Ethno pharmacology"[2].

Resources:

[1]http://www.livestrong.com/article/440673-lettuce-and-diabetes/

[2]_http://www.livestrong.com/article/476862-wild-lettuce-and-anxiety/

Mint

Mint is valued all over the world for its menthol scent and taste. It provokes an invigorating effect on the senses, and is commonly employed in cooking to add flavour to dishes, and as a garnish for desserts. It is also commonly used in medicine, aromatherapy, and commercial goods like toothpaste, soap, mouthwash, balms, chewing gum, and various creams.

Being able to name or recognize all the different types of mint can be a daunting task indeed. According to the University of California at Davis Extension, there are over 600 varieties of the herb. Mentha, Latin for mint, supports foliage ranging from very minute, to broad, and a variety that has a tinge of red leaves. All of these plants come in a wide array of flavours and scents. While the origins of the herb have been lost over the ages, mint is a hardy plant, as can be seen from the fact that it has become naturalized all over the planet in a variety of forms. Below are some of the more common types of mints.

- Peppermint, or Mentha x piperita, is perhaps the best known variety of mint. It is a vigorous herb that yields the classic mint smell when the leaves are rubbed, giving off a distinctive candy-cane aroma with subtle sweetness. It is good for making tea, desserts, candy, and custards. Both the dry and fresh forms are equally good for calming an upset stomach, relieving aches and cold symptoms, freshening breath, and lifting spirits.
- Spearmint, or Menthe spicata, is most commonly used for flavouring chewing gum and toothpaste. This variety is frequently found growing wild in Northern American. The dark green leaves with pointy ends and teeth like edges make for good looking foliage. It is known to drive away aphids, or plant lice, making it a good companion for roses.
- It is the most frequently used variety in the kitchen and makes a good addition to salads, savoury or sweet dishes. Medicinally it acts as an antispasmodic and is good for treating different types of nausea.
- Mentha piperita (chocolate mint) is a close relative of spearmint. It can be easily recognized due to its purple stem with cocoa

165

smell and taste- minus the calories. For people who enjoy chocolate with a crisp mint flavour, this is the perfect variety for refreshing the palate after a rich meal. It can also be used to make teas, or added to fresh fruit, and baked dishes.

- There is a large number of fruit flavoured mints like apple mint, lemon mint, orange mint, and lime mint to name a few. This variety of mints delivers the characteristic menthol taste with fruity undertones. It is good for adding to salads or making teas.

- The Corsican mint has the tiniest foliage among the mint plants, growing to only ¼ of an inch in length. The bright green leaves are ideal for covering grounds and creating a herbal landscape. When the foliage is walked upon, the scent of "crème de menthe" is released.

- Bowles is most commonly used in English cooking. The foliage is medium green coloured with hairy leaves that are circular in shape. It gives off a smell similar to that of apples combined with spearmint. The hairy leaves are not to everyone's taste though.

History of Mint

Mint has existed since the dawn of civilization. The exact history can't be traced, although it is believed that the plant is a native of the Mediterranean, and it was the Romans who were responsible for its spread, as it first emerged in Roman mythology. The name of the species 'Mentha' evolved from the beautiful fairy's name 'Minthe' who was the object of Pluto's (mythological ruler of the underworld) desires. When Pluto's wife learned of his love for the pretty young nymph, in a rage she cursed Minthe and turned her into a lowly plant that would be tramped and crushed underfoot. While Pluto couldn't undo the curse, he managed to soften it by making Minthe give off a sweet smell when she was trod upon. Hence, 'Minthe' became 'Mentha', the name of the entire species that has thrived ever since.

Greek mythology has a different story about mint. According to Greek legend, two strangers were passing through a village and were ignored by all the villagers. No one bothered to offer them food or water until eventually an elderly couple, Philemon and Baucis, offered to feed them. Before sitting down for their meal, the hosts cleansed the table with mint leaves to freshen it. It turned out that the gods Zeus and Hermes were masquerading as the strangers and so rewarded the couple's hospitality with riches. Thus, mint became an icon for hospitality.

Mint has been valued as an aromatic herb since the medieval times. It was used to scent baths, and scattered around homes to freshen them. During the 18th century, mint was used as a remedy for everything from colic to digestive disorders, and it even made dogs bite! Colonists took mint to the New World to be used in teas for curing headaches, indigestion, heartburn, and insomnia. Since mint wasn't taxed, it was also consumed for its good taste and pleasure.

Health Benefits of Mint

Mint oil is rather potent with loads of varied uses due to it numerous properties. Traditionally it was used to treat everything from simple ailments to gingivitis, spasms, irritable bowel syndrome, and rheumatism. It also relaxes muscles, and has antiviral and bactericidal traits. According to some archaeological verification, Greek athletes used mint leaves to relieve aching muscles, similar to the way it is used today in menthol-filled topical analgesics. Mint is a carminative (reduces intestinal cramping) and a counter irritant.

More recent investigations, conducted by the University of Wisconsin School of Medicine and Public Health, indicate that mint tea may be a practical alternative to pharmaceutical medicines[1]. Making tea using one to two teaspoons of dried peppermint leaves and allowing it to seep for five minutes, can help to relieve an upset stomach and ease heartburn. Fresh leaves and tea bags work equally well. It is further believed that mint tea can enhance mental performance and keep one alert. The cool flavour and revitalizing aroma also helps to make one less anxious. Additionally, mint tea breaks up congestion to reduce coughing caused by allergies and colds. It behaves like an expectorant and aids in relieving dry coughs and sore throats. Finally, it eliminates bad breath due to smoking, eating onions or garlic, and drinking alcohol.

Nutritional Value of Mint

Mint is particularly rich in vitamin C and carotenes. Carotenes give plants their distinctive colours and are precursors to vitamin A. Beta-carotene is the best type of carotenes for human health. It has been shown to be beneficial for eye health and cardiovascular disease. A one hundred gram serving of mint provides 1620 micrograms of beta-carotenes. There are also 27 milligrams of vitamin C in a 100 gram serving of mint. Vitamin C is good for the immune system and repair of tissue. It is also associated with protection against certain types of cancer, like colon and rectal.

Mint also provides many essential minerals such as magnesium, copper, iron, potassium, and calcium. Calcium and magnesium are essential for bone health, and 100 grams of mint contain 60 milligrams of magnesium and 200 milligrams of calcium. Iron is a necessary element of the red blood cells, required to carry oxygen to all parts of the body. There are 15.6 milligrams of iron in every 100 grams of mint. The presence of vitamin C enhances absorption of iron by the body.

Mint leaves are beneficial for the skin, something not many people consider. They contain menthol which helps to increase the flow of blood to an area. It may also stop the growth of a skin pathogen known as staphylococcus aureus by nourishing the skin. Mint has been found to aid in the treatment of herpes simplex lesions. The essential oil in mint is a natural astringent, meaning it will shrink pores giving the skin a tighter feel and more youthful appearance. Mint leaves contain salicylic acid which is an exfoliate that gets rid of dead skin cells and opens pores. For this very reason, mint leaves can aide with acne treatment. Mixed with yogurt and oatmeal, mint leaves make an excellent face mask.

How to Use Mint

Fresh mint can cool, refresh, and brighten up everything from cocktails, to salads, and even rooms. Mint is most commonly used with vegetables like potatoes, eggplant, and carrots or corn, to add additional flavour. Mint can even be chopped and added to omelettes and scrambled eggs as flavour enhancer.

A few leaves of fresh mint can be added to the teapot to reduce the effects of tannin and caffeine. Sweet mint water is great way to refresh yourself on a hot summer afternoon. Just boil one litre of water and add a cup full of mint leaves. Allow to seep for about 30 minutes, strain and cool in the refrigerator. Now you have great tasting water to quench your thirst and help keep you hydrated throughout the day.

Here are some additional ways to use mint:

- Chop and toss onto roasted potatoes covered in a little olive oil and salt.
- Freeze mint leaves in ice cubes to make a unique drink presentation.
- Dried or fresh mint can be placed in corners of cupboards for a fresh smell and to repel insects.
- Mint leaves blended with lemon and olive oil, seasoned with salt and black pepper, makes for a great salad dressing.
- Allow four tablespoons of chopped fresh mint leaves to seep in one quart of boiling water, and chill in a refrigerator before straining. This mixture can then be kept in the fridge and used as a mouthwash.
- Toss chopped mint leaves into soups and stews.
- Chop excessive growth and use as mulch around the garden to repel insects.

Clinical Trials

Due to the many health benefits associated with mint leaves, there are now a number of studies being conducted to find proof and understand how the various compounds in the herb actually work. One study carried out at the University of Salford, in Manchester England, discovered that mint leaves appear to kill cancer cells[2]. Typically, cancer treatments work by destroying the cancerous cells, but mint works by attacking the blood vessels in the tumour and depriving the cancerous cells of oxygen and thereby killing it. This type of treatment will have fewer side effects.

Resources

[1] http://www.fammed.wisc.edu/sites/default/files//webfm-uploads/documents/outreach/im/ss_herbal_teas.pdf
[2] http://www.nutraingredients-usa.com/Research/Mint-in-anti-cancer-trials

Onion

Allium cepa, commonly known as the onion, belongs to the Alliaceae family along with shallots, chives, and garlic. It was previously classified incorrectly and grouped in the Amaryllidaceae family, whose members include daffodils, amaryllis and various other plants with bulbs. The onion plant is made up of superficial roots attached to a bulb, and has green tube-like leaves extending out of the bulb. The bulb is composed of numerous concentric leaves that act as storage for food. The bulbs come in many shapes and colours. As the onion plant becomes mature, it generates a seed stalk at the end from where bluish or white flowers grow in a circular cluster known as the umbel. Some varieties or onions also produce tiny bulblike formations referred to as the bulbils.

White, Spanish (yellow), and red are the three main varieties of onions cultivated. These varieties vary in shape, size, colour, and pungency. Numerous new hybrid variations have been developed with reduced amounts of the sulphuric compounds. It is the sulphuric compounds that are responsible for giving onions their sharp flavour and making the eyes sting. The sharp tasting varieties lose their flavour upon cooking as the sulphuric compounds are broken down. Cooked onions may actually end up tasting sweeter than the new sweet varieties developed for raw consumption.

Green onions are called scallions or spring onions and differ from regular onions only at the time in which they are harvested. Green onions are picked when their tops are still green and the bulbs are less than 13 mm in diameter. They have a milder flavour and the whole plant, including the top, bulb, and stem, are all edible. Normally, spring onions are used as a garnish, raw in salads or sauces, and for seasoning purposes in prepared dishes. Onions can be purchased in a number of different forms including pickled, boiled, frozen, and dried.

History of the Onion

Origin of the onion is disputed as it does not preserve too well for archaeological objectives. Some historians argue they first appeared in central Asia while others assert that they first appeared further west in what is today Iran and Pakistan. What can be stated with certainty is that they showed up in the Mediterranean area as far back as 5000 years ago, as records of the onion exist in the earliest recorded books of the Bible. In all probability, the name onion is derived from the Latin *unus*, translating to "one".

Due to its structure of "circle-within-a-circle" and the spherical bulbs, onions represented the universe and eternal life in Egyptian culture. They were used to fill the eye sockets of Pharaoh Ramses IV when his body was mummified. Onions were also placed in the pyramids with kings like Tutankhamen, to be carried into the after-life as gifts with spiritual meaning. The workers building the pyramids were paid in onions. Indians first hinted at the medicinal value of onions in the sixth century BC, claiming they had diuretic properties and were good for digestion, heart, joints, and eyes. The Romans carried onions on their journeys and introduced them to Britain. In the Middle Ages they were used to treat snakebites and as payment for rent. The Pilgrims carted onions to the Americas only to discover that they already had their own wild varieties. American Indians used onions in their stews. Christopher Columbus presented the onion to the West Indies from where their cultivation proliferated. Now India, China, the US, Russia, and Spain, are the world's major onion producers.

Onions hold a special place in folklore and magic. As a protective shield, onions grown in pots and gardens are said to guard against evil. When carried on person, they keep venomous creatures at bay, and when placed in charms they keep children protected against ghosts. Onions are long believed to have healing powers. A cut-up onion distributed around the house is said to absorb evil and disease. To treat warts, just rub with an onion, and then discard over the right shoulder and walk off without turning back. New England settlers placed strings of onions on entrances to shield against infections, and an onion strategically placed under a sink serves the same purpose. Red onions tied to bed posts offer protection against sickness. In times of tough decisions, placing an onion under the pillow is said to generate prophetic dreams.

Health Benefits of the Onion

Onions have been in existence for thousands of years, and the list of time-tested benefits of this simple vegetable have only grown. Onions are frequently used to avert tooth decay and oral infections. Chewing a raw onion for a few minutes potentially kills harmful germs in the mouth, throat, and around lips. Alternatively, the consumption of equal parts of onion juice and honey can aid in the relief of sore throats and coughing. Additionally, the consumption of onion helps to decrease the pain linked with inflammatory conditions such as gout and arthritis. Onions are well recognised for their anti-inflammatory properties. A mixture of onion juice and olive oil, or honey, applied to the face, is said to be a good treatment for acne, and cuts down on swelling associated with acne. Onions contain compounds called saponins which are anti-spasmodic; making them useful for relieving an upset stomach.

The phytochemicals in onions stimulate vitamin C within the body which in turn heightens the immune system to protect against toxins and other foreign substances that may cause illness. Onions also act as anticoagulants, meaning they behave as blood thinners. The ability to prevent clots from forming leads to improved cardiovascular health.

Onions contain the compound chromium, a mineral which is hardly ever found occurring naturally in food items. Chromium ensures the slow release of glucose to body cells and muscles. Eating onions helps to moderate blood sugar levels, which is of critical importance to diabetics.

The pain from bee stings can be reduced by applying onion juice to the affected area, and is also effective against scorpion stings and various other types of insect bites. The rather sharp smell of onion causes insects to take flight, which makes this vegetable a good insect repellent. A few drops of onion juice can provide relief from acute earache and potentially eliminate ringing sounds in the ear.

Onions are loaded with quercetin, an antioxidant that is linked with inhabitation and development of cancer cells. Vitamin C, another antioxidant found in abundance in onions, cuts down on the impact of free radicals in the body. Free radicals are products of cell metabolism that can turn healthy cells into cancerous ones. All antioxidant rich foods neutralize free radicals. Studies show that that the protective effect of onions is related to *any* cancer cells in the body and are not linked to any specific tissue like breast or lung[1].

A newly identified compound in onions is said to inhibit bone loss in menopausal women, and rival Fosamax, the prescription drug. Onions are also rich in sulphuric compounds that prevent formations of biochemical chains. It is believed that these chains may lead to asthmatic conditions. These sulphuric compounds also aid in the melting of phlegm in patients with severe coughing.

Nutritional Value

Being a member of the Allium family, onions are rich in sulphur compounds. In addition to giving them the pungent odour, these compounds also provide them with their health promoting properties. Onions possess a wide variety of allyl sulphides, including the four most important ones and a wide array of sulfoxides. Additionally, onions are a good source of polyphenols, which include flavonoid polyphenols. The flavonoid quercetin is found in particularly large quantities. Generally speaking, the red onions have a much higher total value of the flavonoids compared to white onions, with the yellow falling somewhere in the middle. Onions are also a good source of vitamin C, enzyme initiating manganese, along with molybdenum, chromium, B6, fibre, folate and potassium.

How to Use Onions

Onions are used in an endless variety of ways within different cultures. The most common use is to add it raw in salads or as garnish. However, some people find them to be a bit too pungent for their tastes. One way to lessen the onion's bite is to cut them up according to needs. That might be slicing, mincing, or chopping. Then just rinse the pieces under cold water for roughly one minute, and for onions with stronger bite, let them sit in cold water for a few minutes. Then spread the washed onion on a paper towel and pat dry. The rinsing or soaking removes most of the pungency released when the onion is cut. The final raw product will be significantly sweeter too.

Caramelising onions is another way to remove the pungency and bring out the natural flavour. All varieties of onions can be caramelised, although some will caramelise faster than others. The time needed to caramelise is determined by the amount of sugars in the onions. To caramelise an onion, cut one medium sized vegetable into long thin slices and put aside. Heat a few teaspoons of oil or butter, depending on taste, and bring to a medium-high temperature. The oil is sufficiently hot when it begins to ripple. Add the onion and stir until all the pieces are lined with the oil. Add a pinch of salt, as it will help to season the onion and speed up the caramelising process. This is because the salt draws out all the moisture from the onion thus allowing it to evaporate. If desired, add some black pepper at this point to further season the onion. Once the onions turn lightly red remove them from heat. The caramelised onions can now be used in sandwiches, salads, salsas, as side dishes with omelette, sauces, and in many other of different ways.

Clinical Trials

Many independent studies and trials have been conducted to understand the effects that onions have on different illnesses. One study, using data from southern European population, found a definite reduction in the risks of a number of common cancers with an increased use of onions[2]. Another study investigated the clinical hypoglycaemic effects of onions on diabetic patients. It was found that the consumption of just 100 grams of raw onions helped to reduce the level of sugar in blood considerably[3]. In a third study, Allium plants, like onion, showed antibiotic action against gram-positive and gram-negative bacteria[4].

Resources

[1]http://preventcancer.aicr.org/site/News2?id=11136&abbr=pr_hf_

[2]http://ajcn.nutrition.org/content/84/5/1027.abstract

[3] http://www.ncbi.nlm.nih.gov/pmc/articles/PMC2978938/

[4] Sivam, G. P. Protection against Helicobacter pylori and other bacterial infections by garlic. *J. Nutr*. 2001;131(3s):1106S-1108S.

Oranges

Introduction to Oranges

Oranges do not exist in the wild; they are products of cross breeding tangerines with the "Chinese grapefruit" the pomelo. They are the greatest grown quantity of citrus fruits around the world. The outer orange coloured skin is known as the epicarp while the spongy white mesocarp lies just beneath. The fleshy inner part is divided into ten or more segments, with very thin but hardy skins which contain the juicy pulp. The seeds or "pips" are also contained inside. The fruit forms from a single ovary and is thus considered to be a berry. Oranges are separated into two main groups, bitter and sweet. The sweet type is the most typically consumed variety.

History of Oranges

Oranges are believed to have originated in Southeast Asia, particularly in northeast India, southern China and Vietnam roughly 7000 years ago. The name 'orange' is believed to have been derived from the Sanskrit work 'Nāraṅgaḥ' and also the Telugu term 'Naringa'. After having gone through different languages and modifications, the ultimate English name 'orange' developed. Historians believe that Chinese farmers set up orange orchards sometime around the 1st century, when nobility showed fondness for the fruit, competition between cultivators led to production of larger better tasting oranges.

Persian traders who traded with India and Ceylon introduced the fruit to the Roman Empire, where they become popular with the military and nobility. Around the first century A.D, Romans established the very first orange orchard in North Africa. Oranges produced there mostly shipped to Mediterranean countries. Soon orchards spread from Libya to Morocco.

The decline of the Roman Empire in the sixth century led to a decline in the orange industry also. When the Islamic Caliphate took over North Africa in the seventh century, trade routes to Mediterranean countries were shut down and new markets established in the Middle East taking oranges with them. By the eleventh century, the orange trade in Europe revived with growers using seeds of Persian oranges imported from Spain and Morocco to grow better varieties.

Portuguese traders introduced the fruit to Europe around 1500, where it was mainly used for medicinal purposes. However, it was adopted for the personal consumption of wealthy individuals who cultivated it in private conservatories and called them *orangeries*. By 1646 the fruit was well publicized and well known.

Spanish explorers introduced oranges to America by the middle of the fifteenth century. Its cultivation was started in Cananeia, on an island off Sao Paulo near Brazil. It is believed that Ponce de Leon, a Spanish explorer planted the first orange in North America in St. Augustine, Florida. Today Brazil is among the leading orange producer, accounting for one third of total world production.

Health Benefits of Oranges

In addition to vitamins and minerals, oranges contain a large number of flavonoids and phytonutrients making them a very nutritious and healthy fruit. They contain a compound hesperidin which combines with magnesium to help decrease blood pressure. The same compound works with another compound in oranges called pectin and lowers LDL (bad cholesterol) by not allowing the body to absorb fats which contribute to rising levels of LDL.

The anti-inflammatory properties in oranges provide relief from pain caused by inflammatory diseases like arthritis. The folate in oranges helps to keep sperm healthy in addition to helping with the proper development of a baby's brain. Regular use or oranges helps to fight cancer of mouth, lung, skin and breast. D-limonene is the compound responsible for this.

There is an over abundant supply of vitamin C in oranges which helps in many ways. It stimulates the white blood cells to fight infectious diseases like colds and flu and builds a strong immune system, while the polyphenols offer protection against a number of viral infections. Working in conjunction with flavonoids, vitamin C also helps to reduce the risk of heart diseases by preventing the hardening of the arteries, like in arteriosclerosis. The presence of vitamin B6 helps to produce haemoglobin which is needed to carry oxygen to varying parts of the body.

Being rich in calcium means oranges are good for teeth and bone health. Oranges have high fibre content needed to keep the digestive system functioning properly. The fibre also works with folate and hesperidin in oranges to maintain the cardiovascular health. The formation of calcium oxalates lead to formation of kidney stones, but oranges contain a chemical compound citrate which binds with the calcium before the stones can be formed. Lastly, the large variety of antioxidants found in the fruit keeps the skin glowing and healthy.

While most people just discard orange peel, they too contain a large variety of flavonnones, and antioxidants. Oranges also contain natural histamine suppressing compounds, which prove to be beneficial during the allergy season.

Nutritional Value Oranges

The macronutrients found in oranges include one gram of protein, 0.2 grams of fat, 3 grams of dietary fibre, 12.2 grams of sugar, and 15.4 grams of carbohydrates in one 130 gram orange. The same sized orange also contains 70 milligrams of vitamin C, 0.11 milligrams of vitamin B1, 269 International Units of vitamin A, 39.7 mg of folate, 0.33 mg of pantothenic acid (vitamin B5), 237.1 mg of potassium, 52.4 mg of calcium, 18 mg of phosphorous, 13 mg of m of magnesium, and 0.65 mg of selenium. Other than these, trace amounts copper, iron, sodium, sulphur, zinc and manganese are also found in oranges.

The white portion of the peel found under the orange skin is rich in vitamin C and pectin (a dietary fibre used as gelling agent). Oranges also contain 20 carotenoids with antioxidant properties which aid in averting blindness after the age of 65. There are 38 limonoids in oranges that are responsible for minimizing tumour formation. In total there are over 170 phytonutrients like glucarates, flavonoids, and terpenoids, in addition to the above mentioned carotenoids and limonoids.

Uses of Oranges

Other than eating them fresh, one of the most common uses of oranges is to squeeze fresh oranges and enjoy the juice. However, care needs to be taken as exposing the oranges to air reduces vitamin C content in them. It is best to consume the juice as soon as possible or to refrigerate it to preserve the vitamin content.

When oranges were initially cultivated, their peels were treasured as flavouring agents, and garnish. Even now the nutritional value of the peels can be employed in a large variety of methods.

- **Natural Teeth Whitener**: a cheap and natural method of whitening yellow stained teeth is to use orange peels. Just rub the inside of the peel over the teeth and watch the transformation. Contrary to popular belief, orange peels do not make teeth sensitive they actually help to prevent teeth sensitivity.
- **Cleaning Agent:** The inside of a fresh orange can be used to clean a dirty sink. Rub the inner portion of the peel against the sink to be cleaned. The oils act like natural cleaning agents to bring sparkle to dirty surfaces.

Make Candied Peels: Candied peel can be consumed out of hand, as garnish, in salads or in baked cakes, muffins and breads. They are easy to make, just follow the instructions below:

1. Thoroughly wash an orange and using a peeler remove the zest of the orange. If a knife is being used avoid cutting the white pith with the orange zest.
2. Cut the peel into thin, long match stick style slivers.
3. Place the slivers in a saucepan of cold water and bring to boil for two minutes to remove some of the bitter taste. Strain and save the slivers.
4. In a saucepan add a cup of water and half a cup of sugar and bring to boil over high heat, allowing the sugar to dissolve. If desired a vanilla pod may be added for enhanced flavor. Add the slivers of peel, allow to get coated with the syrup and turn down the heat, allowing the

mixture to simmer for about 15 minutes or until soft and a translucent consistency is reached. Separate the candied slivers from any excess sugar syrup and allow to cool. Now your candied orange peel is ready to be used.

Clinical Trials

Oranges contain some not so well-known nutrients called limonoids. In human cells, citrus limonoids help fight skin, lung, mouth, breast, stomach and colon cancers. New details of these compounds are being discovered by scientists at the Agricultural Research Service in northern California. Additionally these scientists have uncovered that every time we bite into an orange or drink a glass of its juice, our bodies quickly retrieve one of the limonoids known as limonin. The scientists have found limonin to lower cholesterol. They found that in a laboratory, when limonin is exposed to human liver cells, they produce less apoB, a chemical related to higher levels of cholesterol[1].

Scientific studies show that diets containing fruits like oranges, which have high levels of vitamin C, face lower risks of developing cancers of the stomach, pancreas, larynx, oesophagus, mouth, cervix, colon and rectum, breast and lungs. It has further been noted in these studies that vitamin C supplements do not provide the same benefits as when it is received from fresh fruits and vegetables[2].

Resources

[1]http://www.sciencedaily.com/releases/2005/03/050325185404.htm

[2]http://www.cancer.org/treatment/treatmentsandsideeffects/complementary andalternativemedicine/herbsvitaminsandminerals/vitamin-c

Parsley

Introduction to Parsley

Parsley is a herb belonging to the Apiaceae family, with a biological name *Petroselinum crispum*. It is believed to have originated in the Mediterranean region and naturalized all over Europe. The first part of its name is derived from the Greek word *Petrose* meaning rock, due to its inclination to stick to rocky cliffs and old stonewalls. The second part Selenium is an ancient name for celery, hence it can be thought of as "rock celery". It is believed that Dioscorides, a Greek physician during the early Roman Empire gave the herb its name.

It is a bright green coloured plant that forms as clumps. A biennial, it is roughly one foot tall and almost twice as wide. The leaves may be flat or curled and are held at the end of long stems. The overall shape of the plant is mound-like. During its second year it sends out shoots with umbels of tiny yellow flowers.

The herb comes in three varieties. The crispum variety has curly leaves; the neapolitanum is made up of flat-leafed parsleys with a stronger flavour compared to the curly leaf variety. The last variety is tuberosum which are cultivated for their parsnip-type roots. The roots have a nutty flavor, similar to that of celery and parsley combined; its tops too can be consumed.

History of Parsley

Parsley has been around for a very long time, it was thought to have been used by the Greeks before recorded history. The Greeks even dedicated it to the Goddess of Spring Persephone. According to Greek Mythology parsley developed from Archemorus' blood, the predecessor of death. To say 'to be in need of parsley' was another way of saying someone was not going to survive. It was crafted into wreaths and suspended from ancient tombs, and used to crown Isthmian Games' winners.

Neither the Romans nor the Greeks consumed parsley much, even though they commonly grew it in their gardens as border plants. Its use was limited to chewing so the smell of alcohol on breath could be disguised and it was considered to be a good chariot horse fodder. It was also sprinkled on corpses to deodorize the bodies. Due to its links with death, parsley was used in burial rituals and later in Christianity. It was associated with the Apostle Peter because of his title as a warden of heaven's gates.

Parsley was more appreciated for its medicinal value rather than a culinary treat. It was most probably first consumed in Europe during the middle ages. Charlemagne grew the herb for consumption in his gardens prior to the end of the first millennium.

Health Benefits of Parsley

Parsley has been used to freshen breath since the Roman times but it possesses many other abilities with the power to improve health. If parsley juices are extracted, they need to be taken in moderation as it tends to be a rather potent medicine. It can be safely consumed as a tea.

In a study published in the *Annals of the Rheumatic Diseases* more than 20,000 participants, who were free from arthritis when the study started were asked to maintain dairies. The participants who developed the disease and those who remained arthritis free were focused upon in the follow up studies and it was found that participants with lowest amounts of vitamin C rich foods like parsley had three times more chances of developing arthritis than those consumed greater amounts of the vitamin. Vitamin C serves many different purposes in the body. It is the body's main water-soluble antioxidant that eliminates free radicals from the body. The excessive amounts of free radicals in the body lead to a number of diseases like colon cancer, diabetes, atherosclerosis, and asthma. It also aids the immune system to perform better.

Parsley is a very good source of one of the most important B vitamins, folic acid. While the vitamin works in a number of different capacities, its most vital role is the one linking it to the heart. It is responsible for converting homocysteine into harmless molecules. If homocysteine is not neutralized it damages blood vessels, linking it to increased risk of heart attack and stroke. Folic acid is also vital for proper division of cells making it an essential

182

ingredient for the portions of the body housing fast dividing cells, namely the cervix in women and the colon.

Myristicin, one of parsley's volatile oils inhibits growth of tumors in lungs. It also activates an enzyme that aids in linking glutathione to oxidized molecules that otherwise harm the body. Parsley's oils make it a 'chemoprotective' food, a food that helps to counterbalance various carcinogens. Especially benzopyrenes which make up part of cigarette smoke and charcoal grill smoke leading to cancer. Eugenol is another essential oil found in parsley that has therapeutic value in dentistry. It is a local anesthetic and antiseptic compound for gum diseases and teeth. It is also associated with reducing blood sugar levels in diabetics.

The luteolin, a flavonoid in parsley behaves like an antioxidant and combines with very reactive oxygen-containing molecules and aid in cutting down on oxygen connected damage to the cells leading to premature aging. Beta-carotene is another important antioxidant that is associated with lower risks for conditions like colon cancer and other ailment. In the body beta-carotene is converted to vitamin A, a nutrient so vital to the immune system that it is given the nickname "anti-infective vitamin."

Nutritional Information of Parsley

This very mild looking herb is a potent source of many of the body's vital nutrients. What a majority of the population employs as a decorative garnish is actually a powerful health providing instrument. It is low in calories, cholesterol and sodium, has no saturated fat and delivers ample amounts of dietary fibre, and protein.

It delivers abundant amounts of a number of important vitamins and minerals like vitamins A, C, K and folates and calcium, iron, magnesium, phosphorus, potassium. It is the source of eighteen amino acids, essential building blocks of the body. Additionally parsley contains flavonoid antioxidants like *apiin, apigenin, crisoeriol, and luteolin as well as some volatile oils like myristicin, limonene, eugenol, and alpha-thujene.*

Uses of Parsley

One of the most basic uses of parsley is as a plant in a sunny kitchen window. It not only provides a great source of fresh leaves for six to nine months but also beautiful foliage in the kitchen. It helps to mask the other strong kitchen flavours like garlic and fish. Besides using it fresh, the leaves may be dried or frozen. Fresh parsley only lasts a couple of weeks in the refrigerator, and kept in an air tight container, dried parsley, like frozen, maintains its flavours for roughly one year. The frozen parsley retains flavours better than dried, so if dried parsley is to be stored, it is better to use the Italian varieties as they have stronger flavours to start with.

Parsley is used around the world in a large variety of ways. The Japanese deep fry it in tempura batter, the British make a parsley sauce to go with fish and peas, in the Middle East it is used in tabbouleh (a local salad), the French use it in everything, in the Indian Subcontinent it is used in chutneys and as garnish and the Germans especially like the root parsleys in their salads.

Parsley can easily be stuffed into sandwiches, and chopped into salads. The eye pleasing curly parsley works great as a garnish. A few fresh leaves make a great adornment to any main meal. Additionally it may be added to meats, stews, soups, stir fries and all vegetable dishes. It makes a great supplement to other seasonings or is capable of standing alone. It can be added to dips and used in butter and garlic butter preparations.

Clinical Trials

Much more than just a decorative complement to great meals, compounds in parsley has been found to halt the proliferation of breast cancer tumour cells. A study published in *Cancer Prevention Research*, gave rats apigenin, a typical compound found in parsley. As a result the rats developed fewer tumours and tumour formation was slowed, compared to those who were not exposed to the compound[1].

The oils in parsley contain two components, apiol and myristicin which are active pharmacologically. They might be liable for the diuretic effect of parsley. Rats given doses of parsley seed extract instead of drinking water passed out greater volumes of urine as compared to control rats[2]. A Russian tonic composed of 85% parsley juice has also been used to stimulate uterine contractions for women in labour.

Parsley extracts have shown mild antibacterial and antifungal activity in *in vitro* tests. Furocoumarins extracted from different varieties of freeze-dried and fresh parsley leaves inhibited *Escherichia coli*, *Listeria monocytogenes*, *Erwinia carotovora*, and *L. Innocua*[3].

Resources

[1]http://munews.missouri.edu/news-releases/2011/0509-parsley-celery-carry-crucial-component-for-fight-against- breast-cancer-mu-researcher-finds/

[2] Kreydiyyeh SI, Usta J. Diuretic effect and mechanism of action of parsley. J Ethnopharmacol . 2002;79:353-357.

[3]Manderfeld MM, Schafer HW, Davidson PM, Zottola EA. Isolation and identification of antimicrobial furocoumarins from parsley. J Food Prot . 1997;60:72-77.

Pears

Introduction to Pears

Pears come in a large number of varieties but all belong to the *Rosaceae* family along with roses and fruits like apricots, apples, cherries, peaches, raspberries to name a few. The variety of pears most commonly found in U.S and Europe are known as *Pyrus communis*. This variety has a round body which narrows at the top forming neck like structures of varying lengths.

Another close relative is the "pear apple". Pear apples are more rounded in shape and have no necks, so in appearance they resemble an apple more than a pear, but their skins resemble the skin of a pear more closely. Contrary to common believe, they are not developed by crossing a pear with an apple. They are a separate variety *Pyrus pyrifolia*, and include the Chinese pear, Japanese pear and Korean pear. All inclusive there are over 3,000 varieties of pears that people consume around the globe. China is the leading world producer of pears with Italy and United States following. In the US, Canada, New Zealand, South Africa and Australia a large proportion of the crop is utilized for canning. In Europe canned pears come in second place in terms of pear usage after desserts and perry (fermented pear juice).

The production of perry was established in France after the fall of the Roman Empire and indications of its production in England appeared at about the time of the Norman Conquest. It was well established in England by the sixteenth and seventeenth centuries particularly in west England, where climate was well suited to cultivation of perry pears. In the early 20th century, the perry industry suffered a setback due to the labour intensive cultivation requirements of the perry pears. More recently the industry has been revived with new techniques of producing the drink and giving it a more appealing name of 'Pear cider'. With the revived commercial lease, industry sales have gone from approximately three and half million to forty-six million pounds in England.

History of Pears

Pears are thought to have been used as food even by the Stone Age people. While the precise origin of the fruit is not known, dried pieces of pears have been discovered in Ice Age cave dwellings in Switzerland. In Asia the use of pears dates as far back as 2500-3000 years. Sixth century Chinese writings mention pears growing in the previous 1500 years.

Earliest Japanese written records of the fruit are found in works published in 720. By 1860 over 150 varieties of pears were recorded and the planting of the pear tree was common. They were most commonly planted on property corners to avert misfortune. In Japanese culture the North-eastern corner was thought to be Devil's quarter and the demon's entry point. So having entrances to homes from this direction were avoided, but when absolutely essential, a pear tree was planted as a lucky charm.

Pears were highly appreciated by Romans as well as the Greeks and horticulturists developed more than fifty varieties. Homer called them "gift of the gods". It was believed that pears had aphrodisiac properties and were sanctified to goddesses of love, Venus and Aphrodite. Roman conquerors transported pear seeds throughout Europe on their various expeditions. The most popular varieties of pears today are believed to have originated from south-eastern Europe and western Asia.

Pears were customarily used in Europe not just for enjoying out-of-hand, but were pressed and fermented for production of pear-based alcoholic beverage. Due to the good storage life, they were preserved for winter consumption and grown for livestock feed. Culturally they were commemorated along with the partridge in the Christmas carol *The Twelve Days of Christmas*.

Pear trees were carried to the New World by the colonists and they thrived until crop blights proved further cultivation useless. In the 1800 the trees were taken to Oregon and Washington by the early pioneers and there they thrived in the unique soil conditions.

Health Benefits of Pears

Pears are considered to be a hypo-allergenic with elevated fibre content, but they are unlikely to create unfavourable reactions. In fact, pear juice is safe enough to be introduced as it is mild and yet provides plenty of nutrients.

Pears contain glutathione which is an antioxidant and anti-carcinogenic, aiding in prevention of high blood pressure and stroke. The vitamin C and copper too act as antioxidants and protect the cell against damage caused by free radicals.

Pears are well known for their pectin content which helps to reduce cholesterol levels and has diuretic characteristics, and a laxative effect. Drinking pear juice on a regular bases helps to regulate bowel movements and consuming the whole fruit provides valuable fibre which benefits colon health. Additionally, the fibre is free of calories and helps in keeping blood sugar levels stable. The juice also provides quick and natural energy due to the quantity of fructose and glucose in the fruit.

The folic acid in pears helps to prevent neural tube defects in pregnant mothers, while the boron is good for retaining calcium in the body thus averting osteoporosis. The antioxidants found in pears are vital for the immune system and also have anti-inflammatory properties which relieve pain due to diseases caused by inflammation. The cooling effects of pears are known to bring down fevers while clearing the phlegm responsible for creating shortness of breath in children.

Drinking pear juice in the summer helps to keep the body cool in the heat and boiling the juice of two pears with some raw honey and consumed raw is good for healing the vocal cords and an irritated throat.

Nutritional Values of Pears

A 100 gram serving of pears contains no fat, cholesterol, a trace of sodium and only 57 calories. It provides 12% of the daily needs of dietary fibre, five percent carbohydrates, 5% vitamin C, almost 4% vitamin K, 1% of each of the following iron, calcium, pantothenic acid (vitamin B5), niacin (vitamin B3), vitamin E and zinc. It provides 2% of each of these important nutrients; riboflavin (vitamin B5), vitamin B6, folate (vitamin B9), magnesium, manganese, phosphorus, and potassium

Pear skin contains roughly three to four times greater amounts of phenolic phytonutrients as those found in the flesh. Phytonutrients like cinnamic acid potentially have anti-cancer properties while other phytonutrients like flavonoids have anti-inflammation characteristics. The skin also contains roughly half of the total amount of dietary fibre found in pears. As pears become ripe the quantities of antioxidants increase significantly.

Researchers at the University of Innsbruck in Austria discovered that as pears ripen, chlorophyll (responsible for providing pears their dark colour when not ripe) breaks apart into operational antioxidants in the skin and flesh just under it.

Pears are lacking significant amounts the conventional antioxidants like vitamin E or omega-3 fatty acids but they are a powerhouse of phytonutrients. They include Hydroxybenzoic acids, Hydroxycinnamic acids, Hydroxyquinones, Flavanols, Flavonols and Carotenoids.

Uses of Pears

Pears are great for eating out of hand. Make sure they are thoroughly washed and work your way around the core as you would with an apple. Some people do not like the flavour and texture of the skin and prefer to peel and remove it first. It should be noted that a lot of the vital vitamins and minerals (as well as fibre) are also being tossed out. Another option is to chop them and toss them into your morning cereal for a nutritious breakfast.

Poaching is a time tested way of enjoying pears. Poaching entails lightly simmering pears in water or other liquids until they are cooked but retain their shape. Some varieties like Bartletts, Bosc and Comice lend themselves well to cooking since cooking brings out their flavours even more. Depending on individual taste, both wine and juice make good cooking mediums. Microwaving is another method of cooking pears. Peel and cut a pear in half, remove the seeds and the core. Sprinkle with brown sugar and microwave until tender.

Pear juice is a great way to rejuvenate on a hot summer day. To juice, just wash the fruit, cut in half and remove the seed and core. Press through a juicer with skin. If too much core or seeds are left with the fruit when juicing, it will affect the taste and the juice will turn a light brown colour. This is partly due to the seeds and core and partly due to oxidation during juicing. Pear juice is great on its own, but it can also be easily combined with other fruits or vegetables.

Clinical Trials

One medium sized pear provides fifteen percent of the daily copper needs. Copper is a trace mineral required by the body to maintain a healthy central nervous system. Copper works in the brain to ensure that neural junctions allow signals to pass unhindered. This transfer of signals affects our ability to learn and remember according to studies done by Washington University School of Medicine in Missouuri[1].

One medium sized pear also delivers eight percent of the daily requirement of vitamin K, which is required for clotting of blood. Mayo Clinic researchers in Minnesota discovered that the risk of developing non-Hodgkin's lymphoma (immune system cancer), was decreased by forty five percent in patients with greatest vitamin K intake as compared to those with least intake of the vitamin[2].

Resources

[1] http://www.besthealthmag.ca/eat well/nutrition/5-ways-pears-are-good-for-your-health?slide=4

[2] http://www.besthealthmag.ca/eat-well/nutrition/5-ways-pears-are-good-for-your-health?slide=5

Pineapple

Introduction to Pineapple

Pineapple or *Ananas comosus*, is member of the bromeliad family indigenous to South America. Pineapple develops on a plant that remains fairly close to the ground. Each plant yields only one pineapple. Technically the pineapple is not a single fruit but a sorosis; a mass of a hundred or more individual flowers amalgamated onto an inner stalk. As the flowers grow they expand with juice and pulp to become the 'fruit'. The leaves are found on top because they are in reality the continued growth of the stalk past the location point of the berries.

The pineapple's name arose out of its similarity to a pinecone, but in a number of European countries it is known by some spin-off from the word '*annas*' which is derived from the Paraguayan term '*nana*' meaning '*exquisite fruit*'.

Since the fruit does not store well, it is expensive in countries outside its growing regions as it has to be airlifted there. Adding to this expense is the fact that it has to be picked at the peak of ripeness as it does not ripen once it has been picked, and handled with care. This is why pineapples were a status symbol of wealth and opulence, decorating only the banquet tables of the very rich in seventeenth century Europe.

No part of the fruit is wasted. Left over parts after canning like the skin, ends and core are utilized as food for livestock in addition to making alcohol and vinegar. In places where it is grown, fermented pineapple wine is also produced.

History of Pineapple

The herbaceous plant initially known as 'anana' originated from the area that is now known as Brazil and Paraguay. It was commonly cultivated and constituted a part of the staple of the native Indians. It was also used to produce a local Indian alcoholic beverage. The cultivation of pineapples on Caribbean islands was due to the centuries of Indian migration and trade. Being

191

expert dugout canoe navigators, the various tribes were known to raid, and explore across the huge tropical oceans.

Christopher Columbus encountered pineapples during his second voyage to the Caribbean islands in 1493. It was on the Guadaloupe Island, while inspecting a deserted village, that he saw a variety of vegetables and fresh fruits along with pineapples displayed next to pots of human body parts. The European sailors consumed the new fruit and recorded their observations of the new pine cone like fruit with firm interior and sweet pulp like an apple.

The Renaissance Europe to which Columbus introduced the pineapple was largely lacking the common sweets. Refined sugar was a rare product imported at great costs; fresh fruits too were uncommon while orchard-grown fruits were available for limited amounts of time only. In such circumstances the pineapple with its explosive sweetness when chewed, was received as a celebrity by horticulturists and royal connoisseurs. Despite countless efforts it wasn't until the 1600s that the method for growing the plant locally was perfected. Until then it remained a coveted item which only the few privileged could enjoy. It was so uncommon that King Charles II of England had a pineapple included in his official portrait, because it represented royal privilege.

George Washington declared pineapple his favourite tropical fruit as soon as he tasted it in 1751 in Barbados. While the fruit was commonly cultivated in Florida, it was still fairly uncommon for the general public. It was introduced to Hawaii in 1770 by Captain James Cook but commercial cultivation did not start until 1880. In 1903 James Drummond Dole started canning pineapples, making them easily available worldwide. Production was greatly enhanced with the development of an automated skinning and coring machine making the process of canning faster. Today Hawaii contributes ten percent to the total world pineapple cultivation. Other major pineapple producing countries include Mexico, Honduras, Philippines, Dominican Republic, Costa Rica, Thailand, China and Asia.

Health Benefits of Pineapple

Pineapples are short on calories, do not add any saturated fat or cholesterol to a diet, and are totally packed with health building properties. The vitamin C supports the immune system and fights off viruses that are the cause of colds and coughs. It is also needed for making collagen in the body, which is the main protein used in maintaining the reliability of blood vessels, various organs, bones and skin. Additionally vitamin C scavenges the harmful free radicals responsible for causing of many cancers.

Pineapples go a step beyond and help to fight colds due to the enzyme bromelain. It suppresses coughs and loosens mucus. It also neutralizes fluids to eliminate acidity and regulates pancreatic secretions to help with digestion. The protein-digesting qualities of bromelain help to maintain a healthy digestive tract.

The manganese found in pineapples is a trace mineral required by the body for building bones and connective tissues. Just one cup of diced pineapples provides 73 percent of the body's requirement of this mineral. The beta carotene in the fruit can avert macular degeneration and maintain good eye health in old age. The anti-inflammatory qualities of the fruit can alleviate ailments like arthritis, carpal tunnel syndrome and gout. The copper in the fruit is an important cofactor for red blood cell production, and manganese is a cofactor for the enzyme superoxide dismutase, a powerful free radical hunter.

Nutritional Values of Pineapple

One cup (165 grams) of pineapple delivers 2.3 grams of fibre which is a little more than nine percent of the daily allowance based on a 2000 calorie diet. It also supplies less than one gram of protein and fat and 82 calories, most of which are in the form of carbohydrates. Pineapples are low in sodium, an element responsible for high blood pressure in some consumers.

In the mineral department pineapples are a very good source of manganese and a good source of copper with one cup providing nine percent of the daily needs. Additionally they provide a good quantity of magnesium, potassium and iron along with smaller quantities of phosphorous calcium, zinc and selenium.

One cup of pineapple provides 131 percent of vitamin C, 9 percent of vitamin B6, over 8 percent of vitamin B1, over 7 percent of folate. In addition it delivers some vitamin B3 and K.

Uses of Pineapple

The first step in preparing a pineapple is to remove the crown and base with a knife. Next placing it base side down, slice off the skin while cutting out any leftover 'eyes' with the knife tip. Remove the core with a pineapple corer, or sharp knife, and cut the pineapple up into bite-sized pieces.

A second common way to consume pineapples is to juice them. After peeling and coring, chop the fruit and feed it into your juicer. The core can also be juiced with the softer parts of the fruit, thus reducing waste. The skin of the pineapple is too hard to juice in a conventional way, but it contains many nutrients. The Purdue University suggests that the pineapple be juiced within twenty hours as its quality depreciates very quickly.

Here are some other ways to enjoy a pineapple:

Double Duty Tropical Shake

- ½ cup frozen banana slices
- 1 cup chopped pineapple (fresh)

Directions:

Freeze the bananas ahead of time by mildly greasing the bottom of the freezing container with vegetable oil, so the slices come out more easily. Take the pineapple pieces, being sure to remove any stringy knots as these do not liquefy easily and remain unbroken in the shake. Place a few pieces of banana and a few of pineapples and blend. Note that you will have to use a powerful blender or add a tiny amount of liquid like orange juice or milk to begin the blending process. Add any remaining pieces and blend together for about sixty seconds.

Minty Pineapple Pops

Syrup: Add half a cup of sugar and one quarter cup of water in a saucepan and bring to boil, stirring to completely dissolve the sugar. Boil until about half a cup remains, then remove from heat and allow to cool down (extra syrup can be saved in the refrigerator for up to two weeks.)

We can now use this syrup in the pops.

Pops:

- 1 tbsp syrup
- 3 cups fresh pineapple pieces
- 30 ml of water
- 4 large mint leaves
- Tiny pinch of salt.

Directions:

Place all of the ingredients into a blender and puree until the mixture looks like a frothy juice. Taste the juice and if desired add more syrup according to taste. Freeze in molds overnight for a great tasting snack or desert.

Clinical Trials

Historically the bromelain in pineapple juice and stem has provided medicinal value since ancient times to bring down inflammation, reduce hay fever symptoms, decelerate blood clotting and speedup antibiotic absorption[1, 2]. Additionally studies show that bromelain can be used to manage the growth of malignant cells and tumours[3].

A study with more than 110,000 people found that consumption of three or more servings of fruits containing antioxidant vitamins and carotenoids, like those found in pineapples, reduced macular degeneration by 36%. The three serving goal can easily be reached by consuming pineapples in your salad, smoothie or desert[4].

Resources

[1]Dietary supplementation with fresh pineapple juice decreases inflammation and colonic neoplasia in IL-10-deficient mice with colitis. Hale L.P., Chichlowski M., Trinh C.T., Department of Pathology, Duke University Medical Center, Durham, North Carolina. Inflammatory Bowel Diseases, 2010

[2]Bromelain: biochemistry, pharmacology and medical use., Maurer H,R. Department of Biochemistry, Molecular Biology and Biotechnology, Institute of

Pharmacy, Freie Universität Berlin, Germany. Cellular and Molecular Life Sciences, 2001 Aug;58(9):1234-45

[3]Bromelain's activity and potential as an anti-cancer agent: Current evidence and perspectives. Chobotova K., Vernallis A.B., University of Oxford, UK. Cancer Letters, 2010 Apr 28;290(2):148-56.

[4]http://www.kau.edu/prsvkm/Docs/Benefitsandusesofpineapple.pdf

Radishes

Introduction to Radishes

The edible root vegetable, *Raphanus sativus* or more commonly known as the radish belongs to the Brassicaceae family. The radish is derived from the Latin word *"radix"* meaning *"root"*, while the biological name Raphanus means *"quickly appearing"*, a reference to their speed of germination.

Radishes are widely available around the world in numerous varieties with differing sizes, and colours. They range in size starting with ones that are half as large as a ping-pong ball to roughly 7 – 9 inches in length. Colours can range from red, pink, white, gray-black, and yellow. The classification of the different varieties is determined by the season they grow in. The Daikon, an elongated white variety, (*Raphanus sativus var. Longipinnatus*) which is popular in Asian cuisine is essentially a winter variety. The name comes from Japanese words dai (large) and kon (root), and is a part of every Japanese meal in some form or other. The small, round and red coloured variety, which is most commonly seen in the American and European markets, feature a sharp taste due to the mustard oils it contains and is typically used as garnish or in salads. It is more common in the summer.

Some varieties are grown for the root, others for the pod seeds and still others for their oil. While the root and seed pods are suitable for human consumption the oil is not. The oil has potential as a source of bio-fuel and the wild seeds contain as much as 48% oil content.

Radishes are so well known around the world that Mexicans have been celebrating a festival based on the veggie since 1897 called "Night of the Radishes". For a few hours every year, on the 23rd of December, people dress up and exhibit sculptures made out of red radishes especially grown for the event. Some radishes can weigh as much as three kilograms (6.6 lb.) and become as big as 50 cm (20 in.)

History of Radishes

The beginnings of the radish and its domestication are not backed by any available archaeological records. Evidence of the wild radish, and its relatives the mustard and turnip, is seen over west Asia and Europe, indicating that initial domestication of this veggie took place in these areas.

The Chinese were growing radishes as far back as 700 B.C.E and were responsible for presenting them to the Japanese as a gesture of goodwill. Ancient Egyptian pharaohs cultivated the radishes next, and according to historical writings radishes were used in Egypt even before the construction of the pyramids was started. When the pyramids were being built, radishes were fed to the builders as they were thought to enhance muscle strength and endurance and they were even used as payment along with onions and garlic. Its seeds were minced for oil until olives took over.

The Greeks valued the radishes so much that replicas of the vegetable were created out of gold and offered to the God Apollo. The varieties used by Greeks and Romans were much larger, up to 100 lbs, and these were often stored for winter use. Radishes were frequently served with honey and vinegar.

Radishes were introduced to England in the early 1500s, and were mainly used as appetizers. They were flaunted as remedy for facial blemishes, kidney stones and intestinal worms. While they were not widely grown in the country until Elizabethan times they did find their way into Shakespeare's Play Henry IV - '. . . when a' was naked, he was, for all the world, like a forked radish, with a head fantastically carved upon it with a knife.' (King Henry IV. Part II. Act iii. Sc. 2.)

Colonists carried radishes to the New Land and consumed them for breakfast, lunch and dinner. Towards the end of 18th century a minimum of 10 varieties were being cultivated.

Health Benefits of Radishes

Radishes are recommended as an alternative cure for a large number of ailments such as gastric issues, whooping cough, constipation, dyspepsia, cancer, liver problems, arthritis, gall and kidney stones and intestinal parasites.

Research at the Jawaharlal Nehru Technological University in India indicates that radishes are effective against certain types of human cancer cells. According to results published in the 2010 September issue of "Plant Foods For Human Nutrition", the compounds isothiocyanates found in radishes affect genetic paths of cancer-inducing cells thereby leading to their death.

The vitamin C in radishes helps to reconstruct tissues, blood vessels, provides immunity, and has antioxidant characteristics that reduce cell destruction and cut down of cancerous growths. Radishes are very useful as a treatment for jaundice as they eliminate bilirubin from the body and keep its production in check. They are good detoxifiers and play an important role in maintaining liver health. They also enhance the supply of oxygen to red blood cells, thus keeping red blood cell damage in check.

Radishes are a good source of potassium, calcium and manganese and low in sodium. Sodium is the source of high blood pressure while potassium, calcium and manganese are known to lower it. Hence, consumption of radishes can be good for regulating blood pressure. Since radishes are diuretic in nature, they aid in reducing inflammation and burning sensations that results from urinary disorders.

Radishes facilitate a healthy digestive system due to the roughage they provide. The fibre helps to retain water and cure constipation, and provide relief from piles. Furthermore, it keeps the stomach full longer without adding extra calories, which makes them a good part of any diet plan.

Nutritional Value of Radishes

Radishes are a great source of fibre. One cup of radishes delivers one gram of fibre, and while that may sound, according to the CDC this is 4% of the recommended daily intake. According to a Harvard School of Public Health report, fibre in your diet decreases the risk of diabetes, heart disease and colon cancer. It also provides four grams of carbohydrates and roughly as much potassium as you would get by eating one banana, without the calories! It also contains calcium, magnesium, riboflavin, copper phosphorous, iron, selenium and zinc.

Radishes do not lack in the vitamin department either. It supplies ample amounts of vitamin C. In fact the Centre for Disease Control states that a one cup serving of radishes supplies roughly 1/3 of the daily recommended needs of vitamin C. Additionally it supplies vitamin B and K.

Radishes also produce a compound known as Indole-3-carbinol (I3C). According to a study conducted at the University of Texas, this compound protects against hormonal related cancers like breast and cervical, and it is shows hepatoprotective activity. This means that it detoxifies the body and protects the liver[1].

Uses of Radishes

Customarily radishes were consumed to promote appetite and warm up the palate for food, or as an accessory with drinks. Salt was provided as a dipping for radishes, and at times brown bread and butter were also added. This method of consumption is still good today. Here are a few other ways to enjoy radishes:

- **Roasting**. Slice radishes and sprinkle with salt and lightly drizzle with olive oil. Pre-heat the oven to 450°F and cook for 15 to 20 minutes for great tasting veggie chips.
- **Go French**. Thinly slice the radishes and coat with sweet butter and light sea salt. Even though this adds some fat content, it is delicious!
- **Stir Fry**. To give your stir fries some bulk, add chopped radishes to chicken stir fry with spices of choice.
- **Pickled**. Measure out 6 tablespoons rice vinegar, 4 tablespoons of sugar and cut a two inch ginger matchstick and put aside. Take about fourteen radishes and cut them into quarters and salt with a teaspoon and half of salt. Allow them to stand for half an hour in a bowl. In the meantime, heat the sugar in the vinegar until it dissolves. Remove from the heat. Drain the radishes and add to

the sugar/vinegar mixture, toss in the ginger and marinate in a refrigerator for approximately two hours before serving.

Clinical Trials

Traditionally radishes are known to provide a broad range of health benefits; however, actual studies that support these claims are few and far between.

A vast majority of the health benefits are based on consumption observations instead of actual clinical trials. Increased interest in the vegetable has led to more in-depth studies.

In a Japanese study, radish extract was found to improve blood glucose levels in animals. A fat-soluble radish extract was found to suppress insulin secretion and improve fat metabolism in normal animals while a water-soluble radish extract lowered the blood glucose levels without raising the insulin levels[2].

In a separate study healthy animals fed with a diet of radish sprout for twenty one days had lower levels of total cholesterol, triglycerides, phospholipids, glucose and insulin[3]. This means that consumption of radishes (or sprouted radish seeds) may help to maintain healthy cholesterol levels. Additionally, regular administration of red radish to hypertensive rats helped to reduce their blood pressure[4].

Resources

[1]http://www.livestrong.com/article/17858-nutritional-value-radishes/

[2] Taniguchi H, et al. Differing effects of water-soluble and fat-soluble extracts from Japanese radish (Raphanus sativus) sprouts on carbohydrate and lipid metabolism in normal and streptozotocin-induced diabetic rats.

J Nutr Sci Vitaminol (Tokyo). 2007 Jun;53(3):261-6.

[3] Taniguchi H et al, Effect of Japanese radish (Raphanus sativus) sprout (Kaiware-daikon) on carbohydrate and lipid metabolisms in normal and streptozotocin-induced diabetic rats. Phytother Res. 2006 Apr;20(4):274-8.

[4]Shindo M, et al, Effects of dietary administration of plant-derived anthocyanin-rich colors to spontaneously hypertensive rats. J Nutr Sci Vitaminol (Tokyo). 2007 Feb;53(1):90-3.

Raspberries

Rubus Idaeus (red raspberries), and Rubus Occidentalis (black raspberries) are a delicately sweet fruit belonging to the Rosaceae family. The raspberry plant requires nominal maintenance and provides ample amounts of fruit. A row of raspberry plants ten feet long can provide sufficient fresh fruit to enjoy during the in-season, with plenty left over to freeze or turn into preserves. The plants are perennial roots that produce biennial shoots. They grow during the first year of planting and yield fruit in the second year. The original shoots die after fruiting and new ones take their place to start the process anew.

Raspberries are found growing on five continents with over 200 species. Other than red and black, they are available in shades of purple, white and yellow. The purple raspberry is created by crossing the red and black raspberries, while the yellow one is a genetic mutation occurring in the red berries. Black raspberries are frequently confused with blackberries even though they are very different. Raspberries have a hollow middle and are more fragile, whereas blackberries are larger and have their center plugged in.

Raspberries tend to be on the pricey side for a number of reasons. Due to their softness they are highly perishable, and they also bruise easily making them difficult to ship. Furthermore, the raspberry is a hard fruit to pick. They have a short life in the refrigerator too, but when washed and dried with care, they can be frozen easily enough. This is done by setting them individually on a cookie sheet then allowing them to freeze. Once frozen, simply transfer into freezer bags. In this way they can last for up to one year.

History of Raspberries

Archaeological evidence shows that Paleolithic (early Stone Age) cave man also enjoyed raspberries, and they have been a part of the human diet ever since. However, documentation by Palladius indicates that cultivation did not start until the 4th century AD. During the Hellenistic period (from roughly 323 BCE to middle of first century BCE), raspberries were linked with fertility. In Greek mythology, all berries were at one time white, but Zeus' nursemaid, Ida, got her finger pricked and the blood stained the berries red. According to legend, that is how they have remained ever since. The name Rubus Idaeus translates to "bramble bush of Ida", taking into account both the mountain on which they grew and the nursemaid. Back then, the berries were not enjoyed as they are today. The roots and blossom of the plant were primarily used to make eye ointments, teas for stomach cures, treating throat conditions, and as an astringent.

It is believed that the Romans introduced raspberries to all of Europe, but it was the English who first cultivated and hybridized them during the Middle Ages, thus improving them. While it is believed that the raspberry plant was prized for its fruit, it was more than likely valued for the leaves, which had long been used in medicinal preparations. Raspberry leaves are used in herbal teas even today, for soothing the digestive system and providing relief from menstrual cramps. Raspberry juice was also employed in art work during the Middle Ages as red stain. King Edward I promoted the cultivation of raspberries throughout England in the 13th century.

European settlers took raspberries to America in the 1700s. The black raspberry is indigenous to North America only, and is found growing abundantly in the east. Domestic cultivation of black raspberries was delayed until the 1800s. This was because the red raspberries brought in from England were extremely popular and considered a luxury item at that point. George Washington cultivated raspberries at Mount Vernon, and at the time of Civil War there were 40 varieties growing in the country.

Health Benefits of Raspberries

Besides being absolutely delicious, raspberries offer a number of health benefits due to the nutritional content of the fruit. They are great for helping one to lose weight. The high content of dietary fibre in raspberries helps to slow the digestive process, so one feels fuller for longer, while the trace mineral manganese maintains a high metabolic rate which assists fat burning.

Raspberries eliminate wrinkles like magic. A natural face mask made with one half a cup of yoghurt and one cup of raspberries, applied to the face for 15 minutes, provides a glowing skin and reduces the appearance of fine lines and wrinkles. The antioxidant intensity of vitamin C removes age spots and discoloration. Age related macular degeneration can lead to loss of vision due to damaged retina. It occurs in two forms 'wet' and 'dry'. Three servings of raspberries a day can help to improve this condition.

Raspberries are full of antioxidants, among them ellagic acid, which helps to avert cell damage by countering the effect of free radicals. The flavonoid molecules found in raspberries also have antimicrobial properties that cut down the excessive growth of certain types of bacteria and fungi that can lead to vaginal infections and irritable bowel syndrome. Raspberries also have the potential to block cancer cell propagation in various parts of the body, including the colon. The phytonutrients and antioxidants found in raspberries promote a healthy immune system enabling it to better fight disease.

Raspberries are good for overall female health. Tea made from raspberry leaves helps to regulate the menstrual cycles, and decrease excessive menstrual flow. The teas also help to relieve nausea during pregnancy, stop hemorrhaging, minimize pain, and aid during childbirth. For lactating mothers raspberry tea helps to enhance breast milk production.

Xylitol is a low-calorie sugar found in raspberries. It contains only 9.6 calories as compared to 15 calories in sugar. Xylitol is absorbed more slowly by the intestines and is better than sugar for people suffering from diabetes. The high content of fibre (21% of the recommended daily requirement for men and 31% for women) in raspberries helps to keep cholesterol in check

Nutritional Value

Raspberries are an excellent source of some essential vitamins. One cup of raspberries provides 9.6 micrograms of vitamin K and 32.2 milligrams of vitamin C. Vitamin K helps to heal wounds by aiding in blood clotting and with formation of bone, while vitamin C is an important antioxidant. One serving of raspberries also contains 111 micrograms of copper and 0.82 milligrams of manganese. Copper functions like an antioxidant to avert DNA damage, and the production of red blood cells and manganese regulates blood sugar levels and metabolism of carbohydrates.

Raspberries are one of the ten best antioxidant-supplying foods. Anthocyanins are a group of flavanoids that, besides being responsible for the colour in the berries, aids in the prevention of heart disease and dementia. Pale coloured berries, like yellow raspberries, have significantly lower amounts of anthocyanins. The soaring amounts of ellagic and gallic acids, along with cyanidins, catechins, quercetin, and pelargonidins in the berries, equip the fruit with cancer-fighting abilities. Other nutrients found in raspberries include vitamin B-6, niacin, riboflavin and folic acid which aid in maintaining the body's metabolism of carbohydrates, fats, and proteins. They are also rich in potassium, iron and magnesium. Potassium is necessary in controlling blood pressure and heart rate, while iron is needed to carry oxygen to all parts of the body.

How to Use Raspberries

Raspberries can be enjoyed in a large number of ways, but because they are very fragile they do need to be handled with care. They should be used within a day or two of purchase, and should be washed just before consumption or preparation for a recipe so that they don't become water-logged. Also, raspberries should not be left standing at room temperature for too long or they will go bad very quickly. Overly soft berries should only be used in sauces or coulis which require them to be pureed.

Some fast serving ways to enjoy this tasty fruit include:

- Mixed with porridge for a nutritious start to the day.
- Sprinkling fresh raspberries with balsamic vinegar is a sure way to send your palate into seventh heaven.
- Combined with plain yoghurt and lightly sweetened with honey.
- Make raspberry coulis and use as sauce with poultry dishes.

One of the best and perhaps most loved ways to enjoy raspberries it to make sorbets out of them. The beautiful deep purplish colour and sweet tart flavour is a major attraction for young and old alike. To prepare the sorbet puree, put either fresh or frozen raspberries into a blender with sugar and lemon juice to taste. Blend until smooth, strain the mixture into a bowl, then cover and freeze for a few hours. It makes a great snack or dessert for a summer party.

Clinical Trials

According to statistics compiled by the National Cancer Institute (NCI), colorectal cancer is the third most common cancer in the United States, and the second most common cause of cancer related deaths. Studies conducted at the University of Illinois in Chicago, have found that diets supplemented with black raspberries produced protective effects and obstructed the formation of tumours in the intestine, colon, and rectum[1].

Raspberries contain several known chemo-preventive agents like vitamins, phytosterols, minerals and flavonoids, which helps berries in interceding at all stages of cancerous development. Studies have found that components in berries cut down on oxidant and carcinogen stimulated damage to cells and promote DNA repair. Nutrients in berries are effective against esophagus, colon, and oral cavity cancer[2].

According to the Center for Disease Control (CDC), over one-third of the adult population in the US is obese. This translates into billions of dollars in medical costs related to obesity. Researchers are working nonstop to find safe and successful weight-loss products. One such item is the raspberry ketone. It is believed that the ketone in raspberries stimulates the production of the hormone adiponectin, which gives a powerful boost to fatty acids oxidation and glucose regulation. It also inhibits the accumulation of fats, so this just may be the weight loss product everyone is looking for[3].

Resources

[1] http://www.sciencedaily.com/releases/2010/11/101102131833.htm

[2] http://www.ncbi.nlm.nih.gov/pmc/articles/PMC3246882/

[3]   http://www.clinicaladvisor.com/raspberry-ketones-may-aid-in-weight-loss/article/301586/

Spinach

Introduction to Spinach

A member of the Amaranthaceae family, spinach (*Spinacia oleracea*) is a flowering edible plant. The low growing plant has leaves that approximately resemble a spade. It is available in three main types, the savoy variety with crinkly leaves, the flat-leafed, and semi-savoy varieties with flatter leaves. If allowed to grow without harvesting, the annual plant will develop seeds towards the end of summer with the leaves dying off. In rare situations the plant grows as a biennial plant in more temperate climates however, the best plants grow in cooler climates.

Spinach leaves tend to be tender with a slightly bitter flavour. The older varieties of spinach can be recognized by their more narrow shaped leaves and a stronger bitter taste. The modern varieties are faster growing with more broad leaves, and are less likely to develop seeds.

Due to it being a low growing plant it gets rather dirty and must be cleaned thoroughly before eating, especially the crinkly leaf variety. The flat-leaf variety is much easier to clean due to the shape of the leaf and is the variety typically used for canning, freezing, baby foods and other processed preparations. The hybrid variety with nominally crinkled leaves known as semi-savoy is usually the type sold fresh in supermarkets. This variety grows upright making it less likely to get mud and dirt caught in the crinkles. Due to its high nutritional value, spinach is considered to be a super-food in the human diet.

History of Spinach

Spinach is thought to be native to central and south-western Asia where it is believed to have developed from *Spinacia tetranda,* a wild edible green still gathered in Anatolia. The appearance of spinach in the Mediterranean region is credited to the ingenuity of Arab agronomists. Since spinach does not grow well in hot climates, they developed sophisticated irrigation methods as early as the eighth century A.D. which eventually led to its cultivation in the region.

The very first documented evidence of spinach is from Persia around 226 – 640 A.D. and then again in 647 A.D when it was presented as a gift to China by the king of Nepal. At the time it was referred to as "Persian Green" and was commonly cultivated in the Sassanid Empire. It soon spread through all of Asia and Europe. It reached Italy in the ninth century through Saracen invaders and ended up in Spain in the eleventh century where it was introduced by the Moors. Spinach was commonly available throughout all of Europe by the Middle Ages and for some time it was known as "Spanish vegetable" in England.

Spinach was a common ingredient in Mediterranean cooking by the thirteenth century and an important part of the diet by the fifteenth century. It was especially valued in early spring when it was ready for harvest while other vegetables were not yet available. Spinach was a favorite of Catherine de Medici, a Franco-Italian noblewoman. When she married the king of France, she took her own cooks with her so they could prepare the vegetable the way she liked it. Dishes readied on a bed of spinach leaves have since been referred to as "a la Florentine."

Spinach first appeared in the Western world in 1485 when it was mentioned in a German cookbook, and was planted in England in the middle of the sixteenth century. Thomas Jefferson grew spinach at Monticello but the vegetable did not gain common acceptance until the late nineteenth century. In 1930 the cartoon character "Popeye the Sailor Man" advocated the consumption of spinach, and the vegetable gained popularity particularly among children, who wanted to grow up big and strong like the cartoon character. Today, the United States and Netherlands are the largest producers of spinach in the world.

Health Benefits of Spinach

Spinach is not considered to be a super food without reason. The green leafy vegetable contains a large variety of macro and micro nutrients that are of benefit to health. The phytonutrients in spinach have been shown to slow the rapid cell division of stomach and skin cancer causing cells in lab animals. Additionally the greater the consumption of spinach by adult women the less likely they are to develop breast cancer.

Spinach contains significant amounts of vitamin K1 which can slow down the activation of osteocast cells (these cells can break down bone). Vitamin K1 and K2 convert to osteocalcin in the colon, and osteocalcin helps to keep calcium molecules in the bone. Vitamin K is also vital to the process of carboxylation, which produces the protein responsible for halting the formation of calcium in tissues. This helps reduce the risks of atherosclerosis, stroke and cardiovascular disease. The presence of vitamin K in the body also promotes brain function and a healthy nervous system.

The vitamins C and A protect the body from free radical damage, while the fat-soluable antioxidant vitamin A aids the respiratory system and stops cholesterol from being deposited in blood vessels. Vitamin A is also good for healthy skin as it retains moisture in the epidermis and fights against psoriasis, keratinization, acne and even premature wrinkles.

Vitamins E and C present in spinach along with a variety of minerals act as powerful antioxidants that fight the onset of osteoporosis, high blood pressure and atherosclerosis. It is also well known for powering the immune system and keeping the arteries unclogged. The epoxyxanthophylls, Neoxanthin and violaxanthin are found in unusual amounts in the vegetable and play a critical role in regulation of inflammation.

The folate and magnesium found in spinach are both good for a healthy cardiovascular system while the carotenoid lutein assists in preventing cataracts and macular degeneration.

Nutritional Value Spinach

Spinach alone provides more vitamins, minerals and phytonutrients than any vitamin tablet can possible provide. Actually there are at least 14 various flavonoids housed in the vegetable. One hundred grams of raw spinach delivers 2.2 grams of dietary fibre, 2.9 grams of protein, no cholesterol, 0.4 grams of total fats and only 23 calories.

In the mineral department, the 100 gram serving delivers 10% of the recommended allowance of calcium, 6% copper, 15% iron, 20% magnesium, 45% manganese, 5% phosphorus, 12% potassium, 1% selenium, 3% sodium and 4%

zinc. Spinach also supplies 48% folate, 4% niacin, 1% pantothenic acid, 11% riboflavin, 5% thiamin, 9% vitamin A, 10% B6, 47% vitamin C, 7 % vitamin E and 604% vitamin K.

Finally spinach contains large concentrations of phytonutrients. It also contains some oxalic acid which interferes with the absorption of iron and calcium found in the veggie. However, cooking spinach for one minute reduces its concentration, but keep in mind that overcooking will cut down the effectiveness of other nutrients.

Uses of Spinach

Spinach supplies a great flavour, texture and colour to a large number of dishes. Added to salad and sprinkled with cheese and lemon, salt, pepper and olive makes for a very nutritious lunch. Sautéed and placed over bread with crumbled cheese makes it a great appetizer. Cooking it lightly and then pureeing it turns it into a soup. It can be topped with sour cream for added flavour. Spinach lasagne is a time tested dish, or sautéed and added to the classic meat lasagne enhances the nutritional value of the dish and provides colour.

Steamed spinach makes a good side dish for fish like grilled haddock or salmon. It can be served with lamb, beef or even pork. It can also be served on top of a baked potato with some cream or butter. Spinach omelette makes for a very healthy and nutritious breakfast. Raw leaves inserted into a sandwich in place of lettuce or between chicken and turkey sandwich with slices of an apple yield a gourmet treat.

Cheese and spinach blend well together. Cut up and added to pasta dough, it produces excellent fresh green pasta. Alternatively it can be used as stuffing for ravioli, tortellini or gnocchi. Baked over clams or oysters and topped with cheese and mushrooms creates a scrumptious main dish. These are just a few of the numerous ways spinach can be enjoyed.

Clinical Trials

The German commission recommends the use of spinach for gastrointestinal issues, stimulation of growth in children, blood-generation, appetite stimulation and fatigue. Presently data on spinach shows most promise in its antioxidant characteristics, its ability to cut down on age-linked tissue damage, and prevention of neoplasm formation[1].

Swedish studies indicate that the veggie has the power to make us stronger. According to their study, the nitrate found in spinach tones muscles. In the study, which was published in the Journal of Physiology, researchers' added nitrate to the drinking water of mice for one week, then compared their muscle function to that of a control group. The mice drinking nitrate water had significantly stronger muscles[2].

Another study that started in 1984 and concluded in 2002 found that women consuming kaempferol rich foods like spinach cut down on the risk of ovarian cancer by an incredible 40%. Neoxanthin, a carotenoid found in spinach is accountable for forcing prostate cancer cells to self-destruct[3].

Resources

[1]http://www.naturalstandard.com/index-abstract.asp?create-abstract=spinach.asp&title=Spinach

[2]http://www.rawstory.com/rs/2012/06/25/study-spinach-makes-you-stronger/

[3] http://jn.nutrition.org/content/134/9/2237.full

Strawberry

Introduction to Strawberries

The strawberry is unique in that its seeds are on the outside. It is technically not a true fruit. It is actually an enlarged receptacle of the plant's flower, otherwise known as a 'false fruit'. The plant hails from the *Rosaceae* family belonging to the genus *Fragaria* and is related to the rose just like apples, pears, raspberries and cherries. *Fragaria ananassa* or the Garden Strawberry is the most universally grown species with most commercial cultivators using one of its cultivars. There are many other plant species grown around the globe in home gardens.

The strawberry plant has been around for a very long time and has had an impact on many different cultures. It has been used throughout history to represent passion, wholesomeness and even therapeutic values. To the Romans it stood as a symbol for the goddess of love, beauty and fertility perhaps due to its bright red colouring and heart like shape. Legend has it that breaking a 'double' strawberry in half and then eating with someone from the opposite sex will make the pair fall in love. Medieval stone masons carved depictions of the berry on church alters and cathedrals to represent righteous perfection. In the early nineteenth century Madame Tallien, a social figure of the French Revolution is said to have taken strawberry juice baths for the fruit's healing properties. She claimed the strawberry baths protected her from skin problems. More than twenty pounds of strawberries were used in a single bath. The fruit also ended up in literature as a symbolic decoration on a handkerchief in Shakespeare's Othello.

It not known where the name "strawberry" originated from, but it is common belief that it arouse out of its method of cultivation. Strawberries were grown on a bed of straw and once harvested they were typically strung on a piece of straw and sold in that way, hence a "straw of berries." They were known as "wuttahimneash" by the American Indians which translates to heart-seed berry.

History of Strawberries

The strawberry plant is a native of North America, but its history can be traced to 234 B.C.E. when they grew wild in Italy. Some archaeological evidence shows Neolithic and Iron Age man ate strawberries, but the original wild berries were smaller and blander tasting compared to the hybrids cultivated now. Roman writers Pliny and Ovid wrote about strawberries, while the writer Virgil sent out a warning to children to be on look out for serpents hiding in grass when picking the fruit from the low-lying plant. In the twelfth century Saint Hildegard of Germany stated that the fruit was not fit for human consumption as snakes, toads and other slithering creatures could crawl over the low-lying fruit.

Strawberries regained popularity around the fourteenth century when initial records of its cultivation came to light. The first significant attempt at cultivation was in 1368 in France when King Charles V planted them in the gardens of the Louvre. The Duke and Duchess of Burgundy followed suit at their Dijon estate a few years later.

When Europeans landed in America they discovered that the native Indians were already cultivating the fruit which was of superior quality in terms of size and flavor to the European variety. The hybrid varieties consumed today were not developed until the eighteenth century by crossing the American and Chilean varieties. Cultivation of strawberries started in California in the 1900s and today the state supplies 80% of the strawberries grown in America.

Health Benefits of Strawberries

Strawberries have always been associated with good health. The wild strawberry, roots, as well as leaves have all been used for medicinal purposes. The ancient Romans used the berries to prevent fainting, feelings of melancholy and all inflammations, throat infections, fevers, kidney stones, diseases of liver, blood and spleen. Recent advancements in medicine also associate strawberry with a number of health benefits.

The rich antioxidant content in the berry helps the body repair damaged tissues and neutralize the destructive free radicals. They also provide anti-inflammatory properties which provide relief to people suffering from ailments related to inflammation like rheumatoid arthritis, and osteoarthritis. Additionally these antioxidants reduce the risks of cancer and are responsible for placing the berry in the top eight foods recognized for reducing cancer risks.

The potassium in strawberries helps with regulating electrolytes. It is also associated with lowering blood pressure by countering the effects of sodium. According to the Food and Drug Administration, foods rich in potassium and low in sodium may cut down on the risks of high blood pressure and stroke. Potassium is vital for muscle contractions, maintaining bone mass and in minimizing the risks of kidney stones.

The folate in the berry enhances red blood cell production and prolongs the onset of Alzheimer's. Just three servings of strawberries can avert macular degeneration related to age. The micronutrients found in strawberries nourish brain cells enhancing its function. This minimizes the age related loss of motor skills and cognitive loss. Folates also help to break down homocysteine, an amino acid in the blood that is thought to be a risk factor for coronary heart disease, stroke and peripheral vascular disease. The American Heart Association approves of the consumption of folates for individuals at high risk for cardiovascular diseases. According to the Centres of Disease Control, appropriate amounts of folate consumption can prevent as much as 70% of neural tube defects in unborn babies.

The malic acid present in strawberries can remove discolouration from your teeth, therefore making them a good alternative to expensive teeth whitening treatments. Just rubbing the teeth with a strawberry for a few minutes a day can provide surprising results. The vitamin C and flavonoids in the fruit are a natural treatment for uric acid. Uric acid is a painful disease caused by the formation of uric acid crystals in joints.

Nutritional Information of Strawberries

Just eight large strawberries (150 grams) provide two grams of dietary fibre which constitutes 8% of the daily needs, one gram of protein and only 45 calories. Additionally they have no cholesterol or saturated fats and are very low in sodium.

The fruit is a rich source of a large number of vitamins. A one hundred gram serving provides nearly 100% of the daily vitamin C requirements. Additionally it supplies very generous amounts of vitamin B6, niacin, riboflavin, pantothenic acid and folic acid. This B vitamins act as cofactors and aid the body in metabolizing proteins, carbohydrates and fats. The berries also contain vitamin A, and E and flavonoids like lutein, zea-xanthin and beta-carotene in small quantities.

Strawberries house a good quantity of minerals such as potassium, manganese, fluorine, copper, iron and iodine. Potassium is a vital cell and body fluid component necessary to maintain heart rate and blood pressure, while copper and iron are needed for red blood cells.

Strawberries also contain anthocyanins, antioxidants which give the fruit its bright red colour. Other antioxidants include quercetin, kaempferol, chlorogenic acid, p-coumaric acid, ellagic acid and vitamin C.

Uses of Strawberries

Since the berries become soft quite quickly after being in contact with water, it is best to wash them very briefly just before use and never before refrigeration. Then remove the green stalk by gently pulling it or using a sharp knife. The berries are now ready to be consumed whole or cut according to needs. To attain the full nutritional benefits of strawberries, it is best to consume them fresh. The nutrients in the berry are not able to stand the high temperatures employed in cooked recipes. Strawberries have a short shelf life and should be used within a couple of days of purchase or picking.

The best, and one of the easiest ways to use them next to just eating out of hand, is to juice them. They work well when combined with other juices or on their own. Making strawberry smoothies is another great option, other ideas include making:

- Strawberry Shortcake

- Strawberry Muffins
- Orange Strawberry Salad
- Strawberry Jam
- Strawberry Pies & tarts

Simple Smoothie:
- Eight large strawberries
- 6 ounces of yogurt
- 1/3 cup orange juice
- Honey (optional to taste)

Directions:

Freeze the berries for about an hour if fresh one are being used, or just use frozen berries. Combine all of the ingredients in a blender and blend until smooth. If desired sweeten to taste with honey.

Clinical Trials

It is a well known fact that strawberries carry a high amount of antioxidant power, just how much was determined by a report published in the American Journal of Clinical Nutrition. More than one thousand foods were analyzed for antioxidant capacity and strawberries stood in third place in the capacity to deliver antioxidants to the body[1].

For a healthy diet, the Dietary Guidelines for Americans and the Institute of Medicine suggest an intake of 14 grams of fibre for every 1,000 calories ingested. Epidemiological studies show that adequate consumption of fibre is beneficial for several disease like colon cancer, type II diabetes, and cardiovascular disease. A ten gram increase in fibre consumption can reduce cardiovascular disease risk by 10 – 30 percent[2]. Victor Fulgoni, Ph.D of Nutrition Impact LLC researched and determined that strawberry consumers generally have greater dietary fibre intakes as opposed to non eaters. His analysis of the NHANES IV showed that individuals who eat strawberries had 30% more fibre than those who reported not eating the berry[3].

Just eight medium sized strawberries deliver 35mcgs of folate, or approximately ninety percent of the daily needs. According to analysis of the CSFII and NHANES IV databases, researchers found that strawberry consumers have greater average intakes of folate as compared to those reporting not eating the berry. Strawberry eaters had more serum and red blood cell folate levels and low serum homocysteine (amino acid linked with heart disease) levels[4].

Vitamin C is an established immunity enhancer and quick working antioxidant. While the vitamin can be produced by most mammals, that is not the case with humans. We have to get our supplies from our diet.

Resources

[1] http://ajcn.nutrition.org/content/84/1/95.abstract?maxtoshow=&HITS=10&hits=10&RESULTFORMAT=&author1=halvorsen&searchid=1&FIRSTINDEX=0&sortspec=relevance&resourcetype=HWCIT

[2] http://www.calstrawberry.com/fileData/docs/Nut_RH_Dietary_Fibre_and_Risk_of_Coronary_Heart_Disease.pdf

[3] http://www.calstrawberry.com/fileData/docs/Nut_RH_Association_of_Nutrient_Intake,_Diet_and_Health_Knowledge,_and_Biological_Parameters_to_Strawberry_Consumption.pdf

[4] http://www.calstrawberry.com/health/folate.asp

Tomatoes

Introduction to Tomatoes

According to botanical references, the tomato is a berry since it develops from a single ovary. Originally it was named after the family it was a member of, *Solanaceae*, also referred to as "solenoid" and at times as "nightshade". However the original botanical name has been replaced *with Lycopersicon esculentum*.

Regardless of the botanical name, people all over the world have grown to love this very wholesome fruit. The French call it "pomme d'amour" meaning "love apple", as they believed tomatoes to hold aphrodisiacal properties while the Italians know it as "pomodoro" or "golden apple", most probably because the first varieties to reach the country were yellow. The tomato has become a part of popular culture around the world. Japanese have named a bank after it, and American's have used the phrase "a ripe tomato" as slang for an attractive women.

A universal occupation practiced around the globe involves tomato throwing. The ritual started in rural areas and was adapted by theater goers to show disappointment back in the mid-nineteenth century. More recently politicians have become the recipients of tomato throwers. In the late 1940s, tomato throwing was organized into a proper event in the Mediterranean town of Bunyol, near Valencia, Spain. The Tomatina festival is held in August, on the last Wednesday and has been officially sponsored since 1979. Over thirty thousand people just bombard each other with tomatoes for an hour. The Reynoldsburg Tomato Festival is a little more sophisticated, in that residents participate in tomato contests and consume goodies made with tomatoes.

History of Tomatoes

It is believed that tomatoes originated in the areas of Columbia, Chili, Ecuador, and the western part of Bolivia. The Galapagos Islands situated off the coast of Ecuador are also thought to be a part of tomatoes' native habitat. The original varieties are thought to have resembled the small cherry tomato. Cultivation of tomatoes was most probably done by the Aztec civilization in Mexico, and most likely in the form of a yellow fruit. It is thought that the word "tomato" may have come from Nahautl (Aztecan) word "tomatl" which translates to "the swelling fruit."

The Spanish explorers and colonizers carried the seeds from Mexico in the 1500s and introduced them to populations of Europe. While the use of the fruit spread in the area at this time, tomatoes did not gain much popularity as they were considered not fit for eating. This was most probably due to the status of the tomato plant being a nightshade plant and being potentially poisonous. At the time, tomatoes did belong to the Solanaceae family, just like potatoes, hot peppers, cayenne, paprika, eggplant and pimentos. Additionally tomatoes contain alkaloids, materials that in the smallest of doses can cause harmful reactions in people with sensitivities, but alkaloids are tolerated by most people around the world.

It was the French botanist Tournefort who offered the Latin botanical name, *Lycopersicon esculentum* for the tomato. It translates to "wolfpeach"; peach to denote its round and luscious appearance, and wolf from its erroneous label of being poisonous. Actually the botanist, again by mistake, took the tomato to be Galen's wolfpeach of the 3rd century writings in which poison packed in food was used to destroy wild wolves.

Today 130 million tons of tomatoes are enjoyed the world over. China is the largest tomato producing Country followed by U.S, Turkey, Italy and India.

Benefits of the Tomatoes

Health benefits of tomatoes have been known for quite some time now. More recently their benefits have only been further clarified with scientific research. Tomatoes contain large quantities of lycopene, an antioxidant known for hunting out cancer causing free radicals. Unlike most nutrients which do not survive the heat during processing, lycopene benefits can even be obtained from processed products like ketchup. Lycopene protects the body against prostate, cervical, stomach, rectum, pharynx, esophageal cancers as well as breast and mouth cancers. Another well known antioxidant protecting the body from free radical and found in tomatoes in ample quantity is vitamin C.

According to the November 2010 issue of "American Journal of Lifestyle Medicine" the lycopene in tomatoes shields bones from damage leading to low bone mass. The substantial amounts of vitamin K and calcium in tomatoes work in conjunction with lycopene to ward off osteoporosis.

The "Singapore Medical Journal" in May 2007 reported that the antioxidants found in tomatoes are particularly good at preventing damage to arteries of the heart. Consuming tomatoes lowers LDL (bad cholesterol) and triglycerides in the blood thus preventing their deposits and build-up in arteries leading to cardiovascular diseases. It is further stated that cooking tomatoes only helps to release more of these antioxidants.

Eating tomatoes can help to reduce the effects of cigarette smoke. Coumaric acid and chlorogenic acid are two components found in tomatoes which fight nitrosamines produced by the body and are the foremost carcinogens in cigarettes. The high levels of vitamin A in tomatoes help cut down on the effects of carcinogens and offers protection against lung cancer. Additionally, vitamin A helps in preventing night-blindness, macular degeneration and improves vision.

The fibre in tomatoes helps to maintain the health of the digestive system by preventing constipation and diarrhea. The fibre content stimulates the intestine's peristaltic motion keeping the digestive system functioning smoothly. It removes the toxins in the body and prevents jaundice.

The high levels of potassium in tomatoes help prevent hypertension by reducing the tension in blood vessels and increase circulation thus reducing the stress on the heart.

Lastly, regular use of tomatoes dissolves gallstones and reduces urinary tract infections. The high water content in tomatoes stimulates urination, and rids the body of toxins including excess uric acid, and salts. Topical application of tomatoes cuts down on the effects of sunburns and eating them protects the skin from erythema caused by UV absorption.

Nutritional Value of Tomatoes

Tomatoes are loaded with nutrients and therefore provide many health benefits. They contain very high amounts of vitamins A, C and K and high amounts of folate, thiamine and vitamin B6. In the mineral department, tomatoes contain significant amounts of potassium, manganese, phosphorous, magnesium and copper. All this is topped off with protein and dietary fibre.

Tomatoes are off the charts when it comes to the phytonutrients they contain. They are loaded with Flavonones, Flavonols, Hydroxycinnamic acids, Carotenoids, Glycosides, and Fatty acid derivatives.

Uses of Tomato

Tomatoes can be used in and endless variety of ways, only limited by one's imagination. You can roast, stew, sauté, poach, or pickle tomatoes. Of course, no one can forget their use in pizza or salsa. Here are a few more serving ideas:

- Add them to bean and vegetable soup
- Add them to an Italian salad with onions, mozzarella cheese, olives and drizzled with lemon and olive oil.
- Puree them with cucumbers, bell peppers and scallions in a food processor. Add seasonings of choice and use in soups.
- Use slices in sandwiches

When you are over run with tomatoes there are a number of ways to preserve them for future use.

- To stew tomatoes remove the skin by placing them in boiling water for about 20 seconds, then placing them in ice water so they are easier to handle. Cut the tomatoes in wedges, and add butter, sliced onion, green pepper, some sugar, salt and pepper into a pot and cook over low heat for several hours. This can be used as a side dish or frozen in portions for use in soups.

- To make a great tomato "juice", remove any spotted areas. Cut into quarters and simmer for half an hour or until tender. Then press through a food mill, or a strainer. Chill before serving.
- To make tomato paste, blend tomatoes in a food processor and cook over a medium heat until they are reduced by half. This may be used in any recipe that requires tomato paste and the extra can be frozen for future use.

Clinical Trials

Researchers at the National Centre for Food Safety & Technology, Illinois Institute of Technology and ConAgra Foods, Inc., found that the lycopene in tomatoes, along with other protective properties like anti-thrombotic and anti-inflammatory functions, helped to lower the risks of certain cancers. They are also beneficial in other conditions like osteoporosis, UV induced skin damage, cardiovascular disease, and cognitive degradation[1].

In some recent studies, elevated plasma homocysteine levels have been shown to be a risk factor in conditions like atherosclerosis, cerebrovascular disease and peripheral vascular disease. Use of tomato extract was found to lower this threat[2].

In recent years it has been found that blood platelets play a role in the inflammatory process of atherogenesis. Inhibition of platelet function (aggregation or adhesion to endothelial cells) can help to prevent atherothrombosis, which is a leading cause of cardiovascular morbidity. While inhibition can be achieved with antiplatelet medications, use of tomatoes has also been found to be beneficial[3].

Resources

[1] SAGE Publications. "Health benefits of eating tomatoes emerge." *ScienceDaily*, 7 Mar. 2011. Web. 18 Dec. 2013.

[2] http://www.omicsonline.org/2155-9600/2155-9600-3-200.php?aid=12200

[3] http://www.spandidos-publications.com/etm/3/4/577

Turmeric

Introduction to Turmeric

Turmeric (*Curcuma longa*) is a perennial herbaceous plant belonging to the Zingiberaceae family like ginger. In order to flourish it needs plenty of rainfall and temperatures ranging between 20 °C and 30 °C (68 °F and 86 °F). The plant is valued for its rhizomes, some of which are saved for propagation the following year. The leaves of the plant are long, oblong shaped, standing about one metre tall at full maturity.

The turmeric is derived from the root of the plant where the rhizomes mature under the foliage. The rhizome is brown skinned with a bright orange flesh. It has a slightly bitter, peppery flavour that is a cross between horseradish and mustard. After harvesting the rhizome it's allowed to dry and ground to obtain the characteristic yellow turmeric powder.

Turmeric has been commonly used in Indian, Middle Eastern and Southeast Asian cooking for thousands of years. Turmeric can be used as a substitute for the significantly more costly saffron, but it is more pungent and has to be used sparingly. It also has a long history of use in Indian ayurvedic and Chinese medicines in addition to being used as a textile dye. Turmeric has only recently caught the attention of western medical practitioners who are finally recognizing the benefits of the spice.

History of Turmeric

While the exact origin of turmeric is not known, it is believed it most likely originated in South or Southeast Asia, probably in the western portion of India. The plant has been harvested for more than five thousand years, and played a vital role in the Eastern cultures. The turmeric plant does not produce seeds, it is sterile. It is believed to have developed by vegetative propagation of wild turmeric and other close relatives. It appeared in China by 700 AD and by 800 AD it reached East Africa and on to West Africa by 1200. By the 18th century it reached Jamaica.

Initially the plant was cultivated as a dye, but later it came to be valued for its condiment value. Marco Polo marveled at the vegetable that had qualities so similar to saffron in the 13th century that he referred to it as Indian saffron, useful for dying cloth.

While the ancient Greeks were familiar with turmeric, unlike ginger it never gained popularity in the West for culinary or medicinal values. It was none the less used to make orange to yellow dyes. In 1870s it was discovered that the root powder turned reddish brown when exposed to alkaline chemicals. This finding led to the development of turmeric paper used for testing alkalinity.

It wasn't until the twentieth century that western herbalists picked up on turmeric. Just a handful of contemporary herbalists recommended turmeric up until the 1980s, and even then for limited use such as a liver tonic or menstrual issues. All that changed in the 1990s when a number of renowned herbalists started to endorse the use of turmeric for a number of major health issues.

Health Benefits of Turmeric

In some cultures turmeric is referred to as "Queen of Spices" due to the wide range of benefits it offers. It provides antiviral, antioxidant, antifungal, antibacterial, anti-inflammatory and anti carcinogenic benefits. The majority of its benefits come from the chief ingredient, curcumin. This component has been widely researched by scientists and is commonly employed in a variety of drugs and pharmaceuticals due to it therapeutic value.

Curcumin is stronger than vitamin C and five to eight times stronger than vitamin E in terms of immunity boosting abilities. According to the University of Texas M.D. Anderson Cancer Centre, Houston, USA, even in low levels curcumin enhances antibody responses. Hence the reported benefits curcumin offers for allergy, asthma, arthrosclerosis, Alzheimer's disease, heart disease, diabetes and cancer may be due to the compound's ability to modulate the immune system.

Free radicals cause oxidative damage to DNA and proteins that can lead to a number of chronic diseases like atherosclerosis, cancer and neurodegenerative diseases. Curcumin normalizes some inflammatory factors like as kappaB, enzymes and cytokines thus deterring the progress of these diseases.

The curcumin in turmeric protects against liver disease in two ways. It acts as an antioxidant blocking activation of NF- kappaB which in turn leads to the reduction of the inflammatory cytokines. In a separate study published in the Fundamental & clinical Pharmacology journal, curcumin was able to prevent and reverse cirrhosis based most probably on its ability to cut down on TGF-beta expression. The study suggests that curcumin may be an effective antifibrotic and fibrolytic in treating chronic hepatic disorders.

According to a Thai study published in the journal Diabetes Care, researchers discovered that people with pre-diabetes who consumed curcumin capsules had fewer chances of developing type 2 diabetes compared to people who did not take curcumin. Drew Tortoriello, a research scientist at Naomi Berrie diabetes Centre at Columbia University Medical Centre states that this may be due to turmeric reducing insulin resistance and preventing type 2 diabetes. He further states that since curcumin is not easily bio-available, it is a good idea to add turmeric powder to food.

Turmeric may help with weight loss and help to cut down on the incidence of obesity related ailments. Obesity related inflammation is partly due to immune cells known as macrophages found in fat tissue in the entire body. These cells give rise to cytokines that inflame organs like the islets of the pancreas, heart and increase insulin resistance in liver and muscle. It is believed that turmeric restrains the quantity and activity of these cells thereby lowering harmful effects of obesity.

Turmeric powder is an age old home remedy for chronic cough and throat irritations. Researchers at Cancer Biology Research Centre in South Dakota, U.S.A found curcumin stifled cervical cancer cells by changing HPV-linked pathways in cervical cancer cells.

Nutritional Value of Turmeric

One teaspoon of turmeric power (2 grams) has about seven calories. It also supplies 8% of the daily recommended allowance of manganese, 5% of the iron,

2% vitamin B6 and 1% of each of the following vitamin C, niacin, magnesium, phosphorous, potassium, zinc and copper. While this may not seem like much, remember these values are for just one teaspoon of the spice.

Uses of Turmeric

Turmeric has been used as a household spice and a home remedy for centuries. In fact turmeric is not toxic even at very high doses. The U.S. Food and Drug Administration (FDA) has done their own clinical trials with turmeric and declared its active element, curcumin as safe. This is why turmeric and its components are allowed to be used in things like cheese, butter, mustard, cereals and other food items in the U.S

In India it is used in beauty products and employed at spiritual rituals. It is also added to canned beverages, dairy goods, biscuits, and numerous other food products. Some other uses of turmeric include:

- Turmeric added to cottage cheese can extend its shelf life by roughly twelve days.
- Sprinkle turmeric powder near your home's entry points to scare away insects, ants and termites.
- Add a pinch of turmeric to creams and body scrubs to enhance glow.
- Add a teaspoonful of the powder in smoothies to get all its benefits.
- Turmeric tea may help you live longer. Bring four cups of water to the boil and add one teaspoon of turmeric powder. Allow to simmer for ten minutes. Add honey according to taste if you dislike the taste of the turmeric.

Clinical Trials

Curcumin is an antioxidant that has received a lot of attention recently. Laboratory studies show that the compound interferes with the pathways of cancer cell development and spread. In rats curcumin has been found to stop the formation of cancer causing enzymes. Additionally curcumin kills cancer cells in laboratory dishes while slowing the growth of the cells that survive, and shrink tumors[1].

The effect of turmeric on irritable bowel syndrome was studied by giving tablets of standardized turmeric extract to patients daily for eight weeks. It was found that the prevalence of the disorder decreased significantly along with the associated stomach discomfort and pain[2].

In a clinical trial with 45 patients suffering from peptic ulcers, the patients with ulcers were given capsules filled with turmeric. They consumed dosages of two, 300 mg capsules five times a day. After four week of receiving the treatment, ulcers disappeared in 48% of the patients. After twelve weeks of treatment, 76% of the patients were free from ulcers[3].

Sixty two patients with external cancerous lesions were treated with an ethanol extract of turmeric (as well as an ointment of curcumin). It was found that in 90% of the patients the smell disappeared with treatment, and the itching disappeared in almost all of the cases. In 10% of the cases there was a reduction in the size of the lesion and pain as well[4].

The German Commission E, which is responsible for determining herbs that may be prescribed in Germany, has approved turmeric for digestive issues. One double-blind study using placebo-controlled methods found that turmeric cut down on the symptoms of bloating and gas in people with indigestion[5]. Turmeric is also believed to prevent plaque buildup that can block arteries and lead to heart attack or stroke. In animal studies turmeric decreased LDL (bad) cholesterol levels. Since turmeric prevents the clumping of platelets, it may also stop the formation of blood clots along the artery walls[5].

Resources

[1]http://www.cancer.org/treatment/treatmentsandsideeffects/complementary andalternativemedicine/herbsvitaminsandminerals/turmeric

[2]Bundy R, Walker A. F, Middleton R. W, Booth J. Turmeric extract may improve irritable bowel syndromesymptomology in otherwise healthy adults: A pilot study. J Altern Complement Med. 2004;10:1015-8. [PubMed: 15673996]

[3]Southeast Asian J Trop Med Public Health. 2001;32:208-15. [PubMed: 11485087]

[4]Kuttan R, Sudheeran P. C, Joseph C. D. Turmeric and curcumin as topical agents in cancer therapy. Tumori. 1987;73:29-31. [PubMed: 2435036]

[5]http://umm.edu/health/medical/altmed/herb/turmeric#ixzz2teUikrbg

Turnips

Turnips belong to the species Brassica rapa. Brassicsa is cabbage in Latin, and rapa translates to turnip. The ancient Roman author used the words 'rapa', 'napus' to depict long, round or flat turnips. According to Middle-Ages English, 'napus' became 'naep' in Anglo-Saxon, and combined with the word turn ('made round') the name turnip emerged. Turnip specifically is a root vegetable belonging to the Crucifer (mustard) family. However, technically speaking, turnips are not roots but swollen stems that happen grow underground.

The Brassica genus is known for housing more significant agricultural and horticultural crops than any other. Most parts of certain species have been cultivated for food, including roots (rutabagas, turnips), stems (kohlrabi), leaves (cabbage, Brussels sprouts), flower (broccoli, cauliflower), and seeds (mustard and oilseed rape). Some members of the genus with purple/white foliage, or flower heads, are cultivated purely for ornamental purposes.

Turnips are biennial plants meaning they take two years to complete their lifecycles, but are normally grown as annual plants. In the first year of growth they store what humans consume as food. If left underground for a second year, the plants produce flowers which turn into seed pods after being fertilized. Turnips are close relatives of Rutabagas, which are actually produced by crossing a turnip with a cabbage. Nutritionally, both are very similar.

Turnips have white or yellowish flesh with a slightly flattened globe like shape. The root is not as dense as that of rutabaga and it's also missing the neck. Furthermore, turnips do not have secondary roots like the rutabaga. The leaves of a turnip have hair like growth on them, whereas the rutabaga has waxy leaves. While commonly cultivated in temperate climates, turnips can resist drought and frost and are easily grown in extreme weather conditions. The small versions of turnips are used for human consumption while the larger ones, including Rutabaga, are cultivated as livestock feed.

The History of Turnip

The precise history of turnip is not known, but it is believed that it originated in Asia and then found its way into Ancient Greece and Rome. Primitive varieties of turnip, and its relative plants mustard and radish, can be found growing all over West Asia and parts of Europe, supplying sufficient evidence of turnip's beginnings in the area.

Turnips had a bad reputation in Roman times, as they were used to throw at people not well liked in society. It is believed that the low esteem came from the fact that turnips were considered food for the poorer country population of Ancient Greece and Rome. The upper class that did eat turnips would always season it with expensive condiments like cumin or honey.

Livestock has been fed on turnips for more than 600 years, especially after Charles Townshend brought them to the United Kingdom. Due to the expense of storing hay in winter months, in 1730 farmers were forced to kill their livestock before the advent of winter. Townshend realized that animals fed on turnips not only thrived, but could be fattened too, and what's more, the vegetable grew in cold, moist climates. Thanks to the turnip, livestock no longer needed to be slaughtered unnecessarily.

Turnips were taken to North America by the colonists and have been in use there ever since. For a large part, initially turnips were managed as forage. Then, in the early 1900s farmers realized its potential as a valuable energy source for ruminant animals. At this time, farmers were generally turning away from Brassica root crops due to the extensive manual labour they required. However, development of new varieties with partially exposed roots made the crops more easily accessible for grazing animals, and so turnips became a more feasible food source for livestock. Grazing animals removed the need for manual labour, harvesting, and storage. The fact that Brassicas grew quickly, yielded large quantities per acre, and easily adapted to existing pastures without much tillage, made them very economical for farmers as well.

Health Benefits of Turnips

Both Turnip greens and roots can be consumed. The greens contain an even greater concentration of nutritional compounds than the roots. Pliny the Elder, the well-known Roman philosopher, regarded turnips as an essential food of his time. Turnips contain elevated amounts of antioxidants and phytonutrients, which are linked to lowering risks of cancer. The glucosinolates in turnips help the liver to manage toxins, ward off the effects of carcinogens, and perhaps even hinder tumour growth.

The anti-inflammatory properties of turnips are thought to be a key element in averting heart disease. The ample amounts of folate (a B-vitamin) found in the vegetable, plays a critical role in maintaining cardiovascular health. Two outstanding anti-inflammatory agents (vitamin K and omega-3 fatty acids) are found in turnip greens. Vitamin K is a powerful regulator of the body's inflammatory response system, while omega-3 fatty acids are the building blocks, and aid in reducing the risk of arthritis, heart disease, and other disorders related to chronic inflammation.

Turnips provide a wide variety of antioxidants which include vitamin C, A, and E, beta-carotene, and manganese. They also contain phytonutrients which help to promote antioxidant activity which fights free radicals within the body, thus saving the cells form unnecessary damage. Turnips provide hefty amounts of fibre which regulates metabolism and keeps the digestive system in good working order. It is believed that the glucosinolates might aid in the processing of Helicobacter pylori bacteria in the stomach. The significant amounts of calcium and potassium found in turnips help to maintain good bone health and avert diseases like osteoporosis. Finally, the low calorie content makes turnips a great addition to any weight loss program, regardless of whether they are enjoyed raw in salads or prepared as a side dish.

Nutritional Value

Due to their super nutritious greens and juicy roots, turnips offer many health benefits both for human and animal consumption. One cup (156 grams) of cut, boiled, and drained turnips provides the following:

- 146g of water
- 34 calories
- 1.11g of protein
- 0.2g of fat
- 7.89g of carbohydrates
- 3.1g of fibre
- 4.66g of sugar

In addition, turnips contain a host of vitamins and minerals. There are 51 mg of calcium, 0.28 mg iron, 14 mg magnesium, 41 mg phosphorus, 276 mg potassium, 25 mg sodium, 0.19 mg zinc, 0.003 mg copper, 0.111 mg manganese, 0.3 mg selenium, 18.1 mg Vitamin C, 0.042 mg thiamine, 0.036 mg riboflavin, 0.46 mg niacin, 0.22 mg pantothenic acid, 0.10 mg Vitamin B-6, 14 mcg folate, 13.6 mcg chlorine, 0.03 mg. Vitamin E, and 0.2 mg Vitamin K7.

How to Use Turnips

While many people prefer to add turnips as an ingredient in soups or stews that are usually consumed in winter months, they can also be enjoyed all year round in other ways. Turnips can be baked, mashed, roasted, boiled, steamed, deep fried, and even juiced. The tops and roots can be added to salads, while the roots may be used to make wine. Some foods that mix well with turnips include apples, sweet potatoes, peaches, lentils, chicken & rice, and potatoes.

Scrumptious Apple-Turnip Salad

1 cup of apples grated

1 cup of turnips grated

2 – 4 tbsp. of parsley finely chopped

1 tbsp. of olive oil

1/3 cup of raisins and walnuts (roughly half and half of each)

Add Pepper, basil, nutmeg to taste

Steam the grated apple and turnips for approximately ten minutes or until lightly tender. Allow to cool off and then toss into a large salad bowl. Add in the remaining ingredients and mix.

Clinical Trials

Turnips specifically, have not been directly used in too many health related studies, but turnip greens have been inducted in several dozen studies, establishing probable health benefits using cruciferous vegetables, of which turnips are a part of. Turnip greens standout as cancer preventing agents. In some studies, the compounds lutein and zeaxanthin found in turnip greens have shown promise in combating muscular degeneration and cataracts[1]. Other studies show that turnips could protect against lung, colon, stomach, and prostate cancers. Studies found that a compound in turnips "induces the death of cancer cells"[1].

Resources

[1]Golub, Catherine. "Be Thankful for Turnips: November Nutrition." Environmental Nutrition Nov 2007: 8.

Watermelon

Introduction to Watermelon

The watermelon grows on vines on the ground. A member of the Cucurbitaceae family, the watermelon shares a relationship with melons but it is not a member of the same genus Cucumis. Watermelons, species *Citrullus lanatus*, belong to the genius *Citrullus*. The scientific name is obtained from Greek and Latin roots. The Citrullus portion of the name is derived from the Greek word "citrus" referring to the fruit, while lanatus is Latin meaning wool-like. This is a reference to the tiny hairs found on leaves and stems of the plant.

Watermelons are cultivated all over the world and having been exposed to different climates, they have adapted over the thousands of years. There are currently around 1200 varieties with different shapes and flesh colour. The traditional watermelon rind is smooth, rather thick and green with shades blended in, while the flesh inside is red, sweet and has seeds. Many of the newer developed varieties are seedless, with flesh colours ranging from red, yellow to pink and orange. Japan has even developed varieties that have solid black rinds and square shapes.

Contrary to popular belief, seedless watermelon is not genetically modified. It is actually a sterile hybrid fruit. It is made by crossing the male watermelon pollen having 22 chromosomes in every cell with female watermelon flower that has 44 chromosomes in each cell. Upon maturing, the seeded fruit with 33 chromosomes is sterile and unable to produce seeds. Seedless watermelon was initially developed in 1939 and became increasingly popular.

In Russia, watermelon juice is made into beer or the juice is simply boiled down into thick syrup similar to molasses for its sugar content. In many hot countries, watermelon flesh constitutes a staple food, is used in animal feed, and in the drier areas it is used as a source of water. In Asia the seeds are roasted and eaten as a snack, while the fruit is preserved by a salting or brining process.

History of Watermelon

The origins of the watermelon lie in the continent of Africa in the Kalahari Desert, where it grows in abundance even today. The locals of central Africa drank the sap of the fruit by just poking a hole through the thick outer layer. Traders passing through the desert enjoyed the fruit and eventually started to sell the seeds on their trade routes. In this way the cultivation of the fruit spread throughout the continent. It is an old fruit believed to have been cultivated as early as 2000 B.C.E. Some Egyptian hieroglyphics depict the locals enjoying the fruit, and it was so highly regarded that it was left in the tombs of kings and queens to nourish them when needed. Watermelon seeds were also found in Tutankhamen's tomb.

Watermelons were introduced to the Mediterranean region by merchants and were known to have found their way into China in the tenth century. By the thirteenth century they were introduced to the rest of Europe by the Moors. They ended up in North America by the way of the African slaves. However it was not until 1615 that the word 'watermelon' actually made it into the English dictionary. The top five watermelon producing countries today are China, Turkey, Iran, Brazil and the United States.

Health Benefits of Watermelon

Watermelon is 92% water so besides quenching thirst, its diuretic character eliminates excess fluids from the body, cuts down on water retention and removes toxic waste from the body. This is especially beneficial for people with urinary tract and kidney problems. In fact watermelons were a homeopathic treatment before dialysis became common. Its fibre content keeps the digestive tract regular.

The chemical compound citrulline found in watermelon converts into an amino acid, arginine once in the body. It maintains the elasticity of the blood vessels and produces a Viagra-like effect. Regular consumption can be beneficial for cardiovascular health. The American Heart Association certifies watermelon as a healthy heart food. Maximum amounts of citrulline are found in the area closest to the cortex in the white portion.

Watermelons contain more lycopene than any other fresh fruit or vegetable. The deep red pigment is found in the red watermelons and functions as an important antioxidant linked with cutting down the risk of prostate, lung, breast and colon cancers. Lycopene is better able to neutralize the oxygen free radicals than even the potent antioxidants beta-carotene and vitamin E[1].

Watermelons are a rich source of potassium which is needed for muscle and nerve function. By maintaining an appropriate electrolyte and acid-base balance, it cuts down on high blood pressure risks. It also relieves inflammation which if left unchecked can lead to conditions like atherosclerosis, asthma, diabetes and arthritis.

Nutritional Value Watermelon

Watermelons are a low calorie food that contains high quantities of minerals, vitamins, antioxidants, and phytonutrients. It also provides a good amount of dietary fibre, carbohydrate and protein. A one cup serving (152 grams) delivers almost 29% of the daily allowance of vitamin A, 16% vitamin C, 7% pantothenic acid, 7% copper, 5% biotin, 5% potassium, 4% vitamin B1, 4% vitamin B6, and 4% magnesium. Additionally it contains trace amounts of manganese, iron, phosphorus and zinc.

Other micronutrients found in the fruit include lycopene in significant amounts, as well as beta-carotene, cryptoxanthin, lutein and zeaxanthin.

Uses of Watermelon

Watermelon is a versatile fruit that may be consumed fresh, in salads, combined with cheese, especially as a compliment to feta and fresh goat cheese. It may be used to prepare jams, jellies, or juiced. Its juice may be consumed straight or by combining with other fruits or vegetables. It may be fermented to produce watermelon beer or used to add flavour to vodka, liqueur or punch.

Some quick serving ideas include:

- Place kiwi, cantaloupe and watermelon in a jug and purée. Add a little plain yogurt and give a final swirl. Serve on a hot summer day as a refreshing cold soup.
- Roasted watermelon seeds can be baked in muffins or breads, eaten out of hand as a nutritious snack or added to cereals.
- The fruit rind can be marinated, pickled or candied.
- In combination with salt, black pepper and thinly sliced red onion, watermelon makes a fantastic salad.
- Watermelon makes a great addition to fruit salad. Fruit salad may be prepared well in advance as the chilled fruit retains it nutrients for up to 6 days.

Fruits like watermelon, cucumber and celery, with their high water content, have a diuretic effect. This means they help eliminate excess water retained in the body. Actually cucumber water is frequently served as a refresher at many elite spas.

Watermelon – Cucumber Slush
Ingredients:

- ½ cucumber, peeled and cut up
- 2 cups watermelon cubes (seedless)
- 1/8 cup fresh mint leaves (loose packing)
- 1 tablespoons sugar
- 1 tablespoon lime juice
- Pinch of salt
- 2 cups ice cubes

Directions

- Combine all the ingredients in a blender except the ice cubes and puree until smooth. Strain the mixture using a fine wire-mesh sieve and discard the solids.
- Now place the watermelon mixture back into the blender add the ice cubes, process until slushy, and serve immediately.

Watermelon juice is a super healing food, especially considering that you can juice the entire fruit inclusive of seeds, rind and flesh. All parts of the fruit offer immense benefits. Actually, if you look at the parts individually, the most nutrient rich portion of the melon is the rind while seeds hold beneficial fat. Using the whole fruit is far better as it reduces the sugar content that you would ordinarily get by consuming the flesh only. So drink up!

Clinical Trials

In a study published in the Journal of Agricultural Food and Chemistry, participants in a study were given 500 ml of watermelon juice, or watermelon juice with additional citrulline, or placebo drinks one hour before working out. According to the results of the study, the watermelon juice decreased the participants' heat rate and muscle soreness the following day[2]. According to the study the natural juice worked just as well as the juice with additional citrulline. The researchers discovered that more citrulline can be absorbed from the natural juice than from supplements. Watermelon's content of amino acid l-citrulline relaxes the blood vessels and improves blood circulation in the body. This same compound produces a Viagra-like effect in the body which might even increase libido[3].

In a study with postmenopausal women, it was found that after using commercial watermelon extract supplements containing citrulline and arginine for six weeks, the women showed improvement in cardiovascular health[4]. Additionally researchers at Florida State University found watermelon to be effective for preventing pre-hypertension which can develop into cardiovascular disease[5]. Pre-hypertension is a major risk factor for a number of serious health hazards like heart attack or stroke.

University of Kentucky researchers have shown that regular consumption of watermelon juice can significantly reduce the deposits of artery-clotting plaque by altering blood lipids and lowering belly fat build up. Hardening of the arteries or atherosclerosis is a major contributor to heart attacks. Addition of watermelon to the daily diet can help in weight management program along with cutting down the risks of coronary plaque build-up and heart disease[6].

Resources

[1] Archives of Biochemistry and Biophysics in 1989

[2]http://pubs.acs.org/doi/abs/10.1021/jf400964r

[3]http://www.sciencedaily.com/releases/2008/06/080630165707.htm

[4]http://www.ncbi.nlm.nih.gov/pubmed/23615650

[5]

http://www.medicalnewstoday.com/articles/266886.php#Watermelon%27s%20
nutritional%20profile

[6] http://www.naturalnews.com/034140_watermelons_abdominal_fat.html

Wheatgrass

Introduction to Wheatgrass

Triticum aestivum (wheatgrass) is typically sold in tablet, liquid or capsule form as a dietary supplement. It is also frequently employed in juicing, as an addition to smoothies or used to make tea. It belongs to the family Poaceae and is the very young grass, between seven to eleven inches in height, of the wheat plant. The plant grows in temperate regions of most parts of the world. Many people grow their own wheatgrass by placing wheat seeds in water and harvesting the leaves. The grass can be grown indoors or outside.

Wheatgrass has a somewhat sweet flavor.

History of Wheatgrass

Use of wheatgrass can be traced all the way back to the ancient Egyptians over 5000 years ago, and maybe even to Mesopotamian civilizations. It is claimed that Egyptians believed the young wheat blades were good for their health. They even held the blades to be sacred.

In the early 1900s, Edmund Bordeaux Szekely came across an ancient biblical manuscript that he translated. He was so captivated with what he read that he formed the Biogenic Society and published and sold the translated works in the form of small books called "The Essene Gospel of Peace." The main concept in the first book was "don't kill your food by cooking it". The main teaching of the fourth book was "all grasses are good for man and wheatgrass is the perfect food".

However, it wasn't until 1930s that the Western World discovered the potential benefits of wheatgrass. Charles F. Schnabel carried out experiments in an effort to popularize the plant and by the 1940s marketed cans of Schnabel's powdered grass in U.S and Canada.

Ann Wigmore was a Lithuanian who moved to the U.S. She had strong convictions in nature's healing powers, in particular wheatgrass. Her beliefs came from the interpretation of the Bible and observing dogs and cats who ate

241

grass when ill. She claimed that a wheatgrass diet had the power to heal various illnesses.

Health Benefits of Wheatgrass

Wheatgrass is highly valued by advocates of green foods as a natural source of nutrients. Its juice is made up of seventy percent chlorophyll. Chlorophyll is frequently called the blood of plants, and is responsible for capturing sunlight. It is also very similar in structure to the haemoglobin in human red blood cells.

Inside the body, chlorophyll creates an unfavourable environment for the growth of harmful bacteria. It can therefore help the body resist disease. Proponents of wheatgrass think of it as a complete food on its own. There are even claims that one pound of fresh wheatgrass is nutritionally equal to 23 pounds of vegetables.

Wheatgrass juice can be used as complementary cancer therapy.

The juice helps the body to build red blood cells, which are responsible for transporting oxygen to all parts of the body. The increased oxygenation helps the body to counter the effects of carbon monoxide and smog and enhance the body's endurance when exercising.

Wheatgrass is also accredited with helping to dispel lung scars and remove toxins from the body. It purifies the blood and increases the levels of enzymes in cells thereby rejuvenating the body.

Wheatgrass has to be juiced for consumption because its fibrous and woody components can't be digested by humans.

Nutritional Value Wheatgrass

A one ounce serving of wheatgrass has no fat, or sugar and it delivers only seven calories. Wheatgrass contains 20% protein while meat has 17% and eggs 12%. The protein exists as polypeptides, which are short chains that can be deposited into the bloodstream easily. Proteins are essential building blocks of the body needed for repair and regeneration of muscle and tissue. It also contains enzymes that rid the body of toxins ingested with the food we eat.

Additionally, it is a rich source of chlorophyll that helps reduce inflammation in all parts of the body.

Wheatgrass provides plenty of dietary fibre and protein. Additionally it proves to be a good source of vitamin A, C, E and K. It also supplies thiamine, riboflavin, niacin, vitamin B6, pantothenic acid, iron, zinc, copper, manganese and selenium. Wheatgrass is loaded with amino acids in addition to the essential phenylalanine, valine, threonine, tryptophan, isoleucine, methionine, leucine, and lysine.

Uses of Wheatgrass

The best way to use wheatgrass is to juice it. Before juicing, ensure that the blades are fresh, free of mould and there are no yellowing sprouts as they spoil the flavour. Juicing of the wheat grass is best carried out in single or twin gear juicers, not centrifugal juicers or blenders. This is because centrifugal juicers and blenders cause too much oxidization of the chlorophyll. The juice should not be prepared too far ahead of time for the same reason. It is best if it is consumed within half an hour of juicing to gain maximum benefits.

The other option for juicing is to use a mortar and pestle and extract juice manually. Cut the leaves into small pieces and place in pestle, then add a little water and grind the leaves into a paste. Pass the juice through muslin or cheesecloth to strain.

One to two ounces of juice are sufficient if you wish to be healthier or just need more energy. Four to six ounces a day are needed to overcome a disease. Start with one ounce daily and build up slowly to the desired quantity. It is best not to mix the juice with other juices and it should be consumed on an empty stomach. Distribute your ounces throughout the day and take them one hour before meals.

Clinical Trials

Treating a variety of gastrointestinal ailments with wheatgrass has been advocated for over thirty years. It was only recently that a study was actually carried out. In a randomized placebo-controlled study carried out in Israel, some of the participants in the study were given 100cc of wheatgrass juice while others a placebo on a daily basis for one month. The patients treated with wheatgrass juice registered a significant reduction in the chronic inflammation disease of the large intestine called ulcerative colitis[1].

Several patients in a thalassemia unit started to drink wheatgrass juice to see the effects on transfusion needs after hearing about it benefits. The positive reports lead to further evaluations of the drink on beta thalassemia dependent patients. The wheatgrass was cultivated at home in kitchen gardens and the patients drank 100 ml daily. Each patient was his own control. The results were recorded and compared to those of the preceding year. The variables observed were the time between transfusions, haemoglobin before transfusion, quantity of blood transfused and the patient's weight. It was found that the blood transfusion needs declined in patients drinking the juice[2].

According to data, wheatgrass juice might prevent myelotoxicity when used in conjunction with chemotherapy. In the controlled study sixty breast carcinoma patients on chemotherapy were given 60 cc of wheatgrass juice during the first three chemotherapy cycles, while those in control group only got normal supportive therapy. The wheatgrass juice was found to be beneficial.

Resources

[1]http://www.ncbi.nlm.nih.gov/pubmed/11989836

[2]http://www.ncbi.nlm.nih.gov/pubmed/15297687

[3]http://www.ncbi.nlm.nih.gov/pubmed/17571966

More Information

Thank you for reading my book.

If you enjoyed this book, please consider leaving a review on Amazon.

You can find the book by searching for: B00JVPLDV0

You can also find more from me over at my website where I focus on good nutrition and health. My website is at JuicingTheRainbow.com

Made in the USA
Middletown, DE
01 August 2020